P9-CEI-978

CONTENTS

FOREWORD

W̲E HAVE A SIGN IN OUR OFFICE that reads, "Early weaning is
not recommended for babies." Although timely weaning is
the ideal, we realize that the ideal is not achievable for many families. *Weaning* is not a negative term. It does not mean a loss or detach-
ment from a relationship, but rather a *passage* from one relationship to
another. Our first three infants were weaned before their time. We were
young and uninformed parents. We misread our babies' cues, lacked confidence in our own intuitions, and yielded to the norms of the neighborhood. We were able to give our later babies their rightful heritage, and
not wean them before their time.

In ancient writings the word *wean* meant "to ripen"—like fruit
ripened to readiness, until it's time to leave the vine. A child's weaning
was a festive occasion, and not because of what you might think—"Now I
can finally get away from this kid." Weaning was a joyous occasion because a weaned child was valued as a fulfilled child, a child so well
equipped with the basic tools of the earlier stages of development that
she had graduated to take on the next stage of development more independently. A child who is weaned before her time enters the next stage of
development more anxiously and is consequently less prepared for its
challenges and less ready for its independence.

An insightful mention of weaning is found in the writings of King
David: "I have stilled and quieted my soul; like a weaned child with its
mother, like weaned child is my soul within me." The psalmist David
equates his feeling of peace and tranquility with the feeling of fulfillment that a weaned child has with his mother. In ancient times, and in
many societies today, a baby is breastfed for two to three *years.*
Westerners are accustomed to thinking of breastfeeding in terms of

months. We would like parents to think of breastfeeding in terms of years. As Dr. Antonia Novello, the past U.S. Surgeon General, commented, "It's the lucky baby, I feel, who continues to nurse until he's two."

Life is a series of weanings for a child: weaning from the womb, weaning from the breast, weaning from home to school, and from school to work. An infant or child who is weaned from these places of security before he is filled at one stage and ready to take on the next is at risk for developing what we call diseases of premature weaning: anger, aggression, and generally disorganized behavior. Over our 38 years of experience in dealing with families, the healthiest children we have seen are those who are not weaned before their time. Kathleen Huggins and Linda Ziedrich make these points (and many more) beautifully throughout this book.

WILLIAM AND MARTHA SEARS
Authors of *The Baby Book*

INTRODUCTION

W HAT DOES IT MEAN TO WEAN A CHILD? *Wean* is a very old word
meaning to accustom a child to a loss of her mother's milk. But today the word is usually used metaphorically; we wean ourselves
from television watching, for instance, or from some other habit. The
original meaning of the word is getting lost in an age when most babies,
at too young an age to protest much, are simply given the bottle instead
of the breast. Since this practice seems safe enough, and often easy, few
of us understand weaning as the great and dangerous passage it is
known to be in most of the world's societies. But when we ignore the dangers and difficulties of weaning, we risk our children's well-being, and
sometimes our own.

Scientists have done little to enlighten us on the subject of weaning.
Most are confused about how to define the term: Does weaning mean introducing foods other than breast milk into a child's diet, or does it mean
stopping breastfeeding altogether? Some writers have assumed that the
two events occur at once, but only in Western society has this been so,
and only since the advent of factory-produced foods. Other writers have
assumed that women in traditional societies were weaning when they
gave their babies small amounts of ritual or medicinal foods. Some researchers have written treatises on weaning that concern only giving up
the bottle, and don't even mention the breast. Some physicians and nutritionists have tried to generalize about all mothers and babies from
studies of malnourished mothers and weanlings in countries suffering
from Western colonization and industrialization. Psychologists and psy-
chiatrists have insisted that weaning methods largely determine personality, and a few have actually compared adults who were weaned in the

early months with those weaned later, finding the early weaners to be pessimistic, aloof, insecure, and unhelpful (Goldman 1948, Slome 1960). Generally, though, psychological and psychiatric writings on weaning are almost entirely speculative.

Anthropologists, including Margaret Mead, have probably been most helpful in developing our understanding of weaning. They have found that women wean at the time and in the way that their cultures prescribe, and that peaceful, cooperative societies tend to have longer breastfeeding periods and gentler weaning methods. Anthropologists haven't demonstrated, however, a cause-and-effect relationship between the way a child is weaned and her later personality. Few scientists of any sort have examined how weaning affects children's minds, either immediately or in the long term. Nor have scientists considered how weaning affects mothers' minds—or their bodies, for that matter.

Weaning methods and ages vary greatly among traditional societies. In some, women don't initiate the close of breastfeeding at all, but let their children go on nursing as long as they like—for as long as fifteen years (Wickes 1953). In other societies, breastfeeding ends in the second year or even earlier, and children may be scolded, slapped, teased, and frightened into leaving their mothers' breasts alone. But both of these examples are extremes. In most societies, mothers don't begin to work at weaning before the child is between two and three years old, and if weaning is abrupt it is also without cruelty (Whiting and Child 1953, 71). The median age of complete weaning worldwide has been variously estimated as between three and five years.

Western confusion about weaning stems partly from the fact that our heterogeneous society has no rules about when and how to wean. In the 1960s it seemed that weaning from the breast would soon no longer be an issue at all—bottle feeding from birth was apparently becoming universal in our society. Since the mid-1970s, however, a far greater proportion of mothers have breastfed, many for longer periods than their great-grandmothers did. Although many women today wean in the first few weeks after birth, often in preparation for a return to work, others nurse for two years, three years, four years, or longer. Preferences about breastfeeding and weaning vary by class, region, and family, but these variations aren't absolute; they are only statistical. Every woman must decide for herself what is best for her and her child.

Our heterogeneous society gives us a lot of freedom in when and how we wean, but also an inescapable responsibility to understand what we are doing and why. Yet advice on weaning is hard to come by, and often contradictory.

From the child's point of view, generally, the later the weaning the better. Babies weaned after about four months are much less susceptible to gastrointestinal illness from contaminated formula or feeding equipment. After eight to ten months, a baby can wean directly to a cup, avoiding the dangers of overdependence on a bottle (see "The Hazards of Formula Feeding" in Chapter 1). At the end of the first year a baby's immune system functions at 60 percent of adult capability, so the loss of his mother's antibodies isn't as dangerous as before. After eighteen months or so, a child is over the worst of separation anxiety; the loss of the breast is a much smaller threat to his security now. At about age three, a child leaves behind the aggressive independence of the toddler years, and will usually wean easily and amicably. And after age four or so, a child can take pride in making his own decision to give up nursing, and may talk about his nursing years with love and gratitude forever after.

From the mother's point of view, the benefits of late weaning aren't so absolute. Whereas some mothers love the intimacy and relaxation of breastfeeding, others complain about being "tied down" or feeling "like a cow." For these women, being physically tied to a child through breastfeeding may accentuate the burdensome nature of parenting, which in our society can be isolating and even impoverishing. Most women, actually, feel somewhat ambivalent about breastfeeding; at times nursing may seem a tender joy, at other times an annoyance. Breastfeeding women may naturally wonder if bottle feeding would make mothering easier. Even if a woman loves to nurse, sore nipples, criticism from family members, pregnancy, or some other problem may drive her to wean sooner than she would otherwise. Weaning may bring relief; however, most women who wean in the early months end up wishing they hadn't.

In the following chapters we will tell you how to wean your baby at any age you prefer, but we will also tell you how to delay complete weaning if it isn't necessary. (If delaying full weaning isn't an option, you need read only the section marked with a colored bar at the top of the pages in the chapter applicable to your child's age.) We will tell you how to avoid overusing or misusing bottles and formula, and how to avoid using these things at all. We will show you that, as long as you are nursing, you can take control of where, when, and how often you breastfeed. We will try to help you see weaning as both an event and a process—a process that begins with a baby's first taste of a food other than mother's milk, and continues for weeks, months, or years afterward. We will try to help you ensure that your baby develops well—physically, socially, and mentally—no matter how long nursing continues. Finally, we hope, we will offer you the ideas and encouragement you need to end nursing not only with minimal struggle and grief on either side, but also with happy memories of your nursing days and confidence in your child's future.

one

THE WESTERN WAY OF NURSING AND WEANING

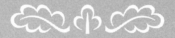

THROUGHOUT OUR SOCIETY, ignorance and confusion surround the subjects of breastfeeding and, particularly, weaning. While La Leche leaders encourage mothers to nurse whenever their children please for as long as they please, children's books show many more babies sucking at bottles and pacifiers than breastfeeding, and children still give their dolls little bottles filled with milky fluid. The parenting guides in our bookstores contradict each other on such questions as how often and how long to nurse, when to introduce solids, whether to sleep with the baby, and when to end breastfeeding altogether. Hospital nurses still may advise a woman to breastfeed, but then give the newborn a bottle while the mother sleeps and hand out formula samples when the mother and baby check out.

Chief sources of the information in this chapter are the following: For "Before the Industrial Era," Fildes 1986; for "The Industrial Era," Apple 1987; and for "The Hazards of Formula Feeding," Walker 1993a.

Medical authorities agree that breast is best: The American Academy of Pediatrics recommends that women breastfeed throughout a baby's first year, and give no other foods besides breast milk during the first six months, and the World Health Organization recommends breastfeeding to two years of age. Still, most doctors are reluctant to criticize a parent's preference for bottles or to question the safety of artificial feeding. When asked for help in resolving breastfeeding problems, few doctors know how to provide it. Many physicians, in fact, openly discourage breastfeeding after a baby's first year.

Small wonder, then, that almost two-thirds of U.S. mothers wean their babies within six months of birth, if they breastfeed at all. An educated few may go on nursing for years, but even many in this small group feel ambivalent and defensive, especially if their toddlers are nursing many times per day and showing no inclination to self-wean. Meanwhile, as wage labor and factory goods, including formula, spread through the non-Western world, women in developing countries are finding their milk running dry.

How did we reach this state of confusion? Didn't our foremothers all nurse successfully for long periods, and didn't they all know how to go about weaning?

That your great-grandmother had a long and satisfying breastfeeding experience is more likely if she was from an African, Asian, or other non-Western society. The most characteristic mode of human infant care the world over, in fact, is much like that of other primates: The mother keeps her baby near her continuously, and she nurses often, as much for the child's pacification as for nourishment, at least until the child is able to feed herself and get about independently. Favored children may be nursed much longer: Pu Yi, the last emperor of China, was suckled by a wet nurse until he turned eight. Of 52 societies included in an anthropological study of child-rearing practices, only two weaned their children before the age of one year (Whiting and Child 1953). When a mother does call a stop to breastfeeding, she usually substitutes tasty, rich foods and a lot of attention.

Among Western peoples, however, a long history of ambivalence about breastfeeding fosters a disregard for young children's suckling needs, ignorance about normal mammary function, and an eagerness to substitute artificial foods and feeding methods for that which nature has provided. It's important to know a little of this history if we are to clear our minds of its legacy—the vague fears and irrational biases that inhibit successful breastfeeding. For hundreds of years, women have been hearing that their breast milk is "bad," that it can "dry up" unexpectedly, that breastfeeding is unseemly and a sign of poverty, and that substitutes are as good as or better than the real thing.

BEFORE THE INDUSTRIAL ERA

In the ancient world, of both the West and the East, women breastfed much longer than Western women do today. Three years was the common age of complete weaning among the ancient Hebrews; later the Talmud specified a nursing period of twenty-four months. Wet-nursing contracts in Babylonia required breastfeeding for two or three years. A medical text of ancient India said weaning from the breast should begin only after the child's second birthday. The Koran, likewise, said that a baby should be suckled for two years.

Breastfeeding was the norm in ancient Greece, too; however, weaning apparently occurred quite early. Wet-nursing contracts called for only six months of breastfeeding, followed by eighteen months of feeding cow's milk. So many infant feeding vessels from the period have been discovered that we can't assume they were all used by foundlings; weaning must usually have begun before a child could eat the food of adults. Aristotle's statement that "so long as there is flow of milk the menstrual purgations do not take place" suggests that, although breastfeeding was unrestricted in the early months, it seldom continued until the time a woman nursing without restriction normally resumes menstruation, between one and two years after her baby's birth.

In ancient Rome, nursing women were celebrated as goddesses of maternal love and fertility. Two Roman doctors, Soranus and Galen, wrote what were to remain until the eighteenth century the standard Western references on infant care. They believed complete weaning shouldn't occur until the child turned three (Galen) or had all his baby teeth (Soranus).

Like later doctors, however, Soranus didn't expect every woman to live up to maternal ideals. A woman of means should hire a wet nurse, he wrote, to avoid premature aging, emaciation, and distended breasts. Soranus may also have been the first writer to claim that crying is good for a baby's lungs, that a mother who sleeps with her baby might bruise or smother the child in rolling over, and that frequent nursing, especially at night, might cause epilepsy and apoplexy (stroke).

Another Roman writer praised the Spartans for restricting nursings to avoid overfeeding: "For when a child is completely satisfied, it sleeps much and becomes lethargic, and its belly is distended and full of wind, and its urine watery" (Fildes 1986, 29-30). The fear of satisfying a baby's appetite, dating at least to these ancient Romans, would peak in the nineteenth and early twentieth centuries, when it would cause widespread failure of lactation and undernourishment of babies in the United States and throughout the West.

Roman women apparently responded to these mixed messages about the value of breastfeeding by tending to cut the nursing period short. Soranus complained that women who were "too hasty" or who found nursing "a burden" gave cereal food after only forty days. That signs of rickets have been found in the remains of Roman children and adults indicates that many Romans were weaned earlier than the physicians advised.

In medieval Europe, although most mothers nursed without restriction, many noble and wealthy women hired wet nurses. This practice became more and more the norm after the eleventh century; in some areas even artisans and small shopkeepers employed wet nurses. Nursing was the lot of the poor, who had no other choice.

Sixteenth- and seventeenth-century priests and physicians condemned the practice of wet nursing; they believed the wet-nursed child would "soukethe the vice of his nouryse with the milke of her pappe," as a sixteenth-century writer put it (Wickes 1953). Wealthy women came to believe breastfeeding would make them look old, prevent them from dressing fashionably, and make their breasts sag. They and their mates also understood that nursing would delay the return of their fertility and so prevent them from producing the expected ten or twelve heirs. From the sixteenth century on, moreover, many wealthy women were unable to suckle; their corsets or stays, worn from the age of two and a half or three, flattened their breasts, which sometimes caused the nipples to become inverted or otherwise deformed. Even if a woman were able and eager to nurse her own children, her mate would likely forbid it. And she would need great courage and resolve to overcome the "unhandsome reflections and bitter taunts from others of a contrary practice," as one writer observed in 1695. "A lady that will condescend to be a nurse, though to her own child, is become as unfashionable and ungenteel as a gentleman that will not drink, swear and be profane" (Fildes 1986, 100-110).

Medical writers, still following their Roman predecessors, advised breastfeeding for a child's first two years, but not all children were granted so generous a nursing period. An Italian physician, Hieronymus Mercurialis, reported in 1583 that most women stopped breastfeeding by the thirteenth month, and a sixteenth-century German physician wrote that in his experience women most commonly suckled for just a year (Wickes 1953). Valerie Fildes (1986, 370) found that children of the educated in early sixteenth-century England were nursed an average of eighteen months. Children of the poor may have been weaned even earlier.

Women's tendency to wean earlier than recommended may have been partly due to the substantial cultural restrictions placed on breastfeeding: A woman wasn't supposed to nurse when pregnant or menstruating, when her milk was thought to be "bad" or nonexistent; she was to abstain from sex through the nursing period (as directed by the Roman Galen); and she wasn't to share a bed with her baby, since what we now call Sudden Infant Death Syndrome (SIDS, or crib death) was attributed to mothers' smothering their babies by lying upon them. Women probably defied these restrictions, though secretly, more often than they abided by them.

Partially to blame for early weaning, too, was the practice of early mixed feeding. Mercurialis claimed that infants were given sopped bread as early as the third month, and meat broth even earlier, to appease them during the long periods their mothers were away working. A seventeenth-century Scottish writer reported that many women gave their children pap (flour or bread crumbs cooked in water or milk) as soon as they were born. Not only the infants of the poor received pap; the future King Louis XIII received it from the age of eighteen days, because his physician thought his nurses had too little milk. Then as now, substituting other foods for nursings reduced women's milk production, so their babies soon became dependent on pap and panada (a mixture of bread, broth or milk, and sometimes eggs or other ingredients), as lacking as these usually were in protein and vitamins.

Weaning was a simple matter for most wealthy women, although often calamitous for their children: A child was simply taken from the wet nurse's home, the only home he had ever known, and returned to his family of birth, or, less often, the wet nurse was sent away from the family's home. Or the nurse might wean the child by applying a bitter substance to her breasts or frightening the child. Among both rich and poor, according to Valerie Fildes, abrupt weaning methods such as these may have been more common than gradual methods, despite the disapproval of medical writers.

In certain areas of Europe, including parts of Germany and Russia, parents of all classes relied entirely on artificial feeding from the birth of their babies onward. Whether this custom arose to allow women freedom as they worked is unknown; in Tyrol the tight dresses women wore prevented suckling. In any case, men and women in these areas considered breastfeeding disgusting. In Bavaria, where the infant mortality rate was especially high, breastfeeding was considered "swinish and filthy"(Fildes 1986, 264). In Muscovy and Iceland, babies were left lying on the floor to suck milk or whey through a tube whenever they were hungry, much as many babies today lie in a crib or car seat sucking at a propped bottle. The cold, dry climates of these areas, along with a trial-and-error learning of sanitary procedures, apparently enabled adequate numbers of artificially fed infants to survive. Since artificial feeding prevailed in these regions through the nineteenth century, when it became commonplace elsewhere, we can surmise that many of our European ancestors came to America believing that breastfeeding is unseemly and unnecessary.

In England in the late seventeenth and eighteenth centuries, when wet nurses were getting blamed for all sorts of infant illnesses, wealthy men began experimenting with artificial feeding. They may have been influenced by the writings of Johann Van Helmont, a Belgian chemist who condemned the use of all milk, especially breast milk, and advised feeding all babies on a panada of bread, smallbeer, and honey or sugar. Likewise avoiding milk, the English fathers usually chose a combination of bread and water. The infant son of King James II, fed on this diet for seven weeks, was nearly dead when his father changed his mind and hired a wet nurse. Less lucky was a son of the Duke of Buckingham, who starved on the same diet.

As far as we know, the wives of these men never supported the fashion of artificial feeding from birth. Wealthy Englishwomen mostly favored wet nursing until the mid-eighteenth century, when they began to prefer nursing their own children. They may have been influenced by the writings of Jean-Jacques Rousseau, who in *Émile* (1762) condemned wet nursing as unnatural.

Women did not, however, heed Rousseau's condemnation of early weaning. By the late eighteenth century, the median age of weaning among educated people in Britain was seven and a quarter months. Early weaning was supported by most eighteenth-century medical writers, who advised only eight to nine months of breastfeeding. Believing that breast milk deteriorated after several months of lactation and actually became harmful for the child, they became intolerant of longer suckling. "Fright, anxiety, loss of appetite, menstruation, pregnancy, sickness, drunkenness and greediness" in the breastfeeding woman were all thought to affect her milk, and so were indications for weaning even earlier than eight to nine months (Fildes 1986, 369).

The wealthy Englishmen's failed experiments in artificial feeding had incited much medical discussion on substitute foods and the widespread manufacture of various feeding vessels—the pap boat, which looked like a gravy boat, the "bubbly pot," a lidded can with a long, narrow spout covered with a sponge and parchment, and the metal or glass sucking bottle. By the end of the seventeenth century, medical writers were promoting mixed feeding at two to four months. Early supplementation and total artificial feeding became common in the American colonies, which had a thriving trade in sucking bottles.

In an era without refrigeration, feeding babies animal milk, or mixtures containing animal milk, was hazardous if the milk wasn't very fresh (boiling milk destroys harmful bacteria, but eighteenth-century parents apparently understood that boiling also destroys beneficial properties in milk—that is, vitamins—and so preferred to use raw milk). Dirty utensils also could contaminate artificial foods. The traditional feeding horn, a cow's horn covered with parchment, was difficult to clean thoroughly, as were the newfangled bubbly pot and many kinds of sucking bottles. The younger babies were weaned, the more such feeding devices were relied upon. Gastrointestinal illness in infants, therefore, became a great concern of parents and physicians. Diarrhea from food contamination became epidemic, especially in warm weather, when harmful bacteria multiplied fastest.

"Summer complaint," "watery gripes," and "cholera infantum" are all old names for infant diarrhea, or gastroenteritis, which is often caused by germ-laden artificial foods and feeding methods. In the United States today, babies fed only formula are approximately three times as likely as fully breastfed babies to be taken to the doctor or to be hospitalized for gastroenteritis (Ball and Wright 1999).

Ignorant of the true cause of the illness, many doctors blamed babies' gastrointestinal problems on overfeeding. Overfeeding, they believed, caused vomiting, distended belly, abdominal pain, indigestion, and diarrhea—as well as nearly all childhood diseases, fever, convulsions, breathing difficulties, and death (Fildes 1986, 251; Wickes 1953). The physicians' solution was to restrict feedings so that the baby's hunger was never satisfied. Underfeeding of infants was so much the norm in eighteenth-century France that the physician N. Brouzet, while pleading for breastfeeding "according to the appetite of the infants," added that ideally two or, at most, three daily feedings would best promote healthy digestion. William Cadogan was the first English physician to promote feeding schedules; he advised four feedings in each twenty-four-hour period (Wickes 1953). Limiting feedings according to doctors' advice must have reduced some mothers' milk supplies, and thereby necessitated early weaning whether the women wanted it or not.

Although babies weaned in poor families, whose diets included cheese, legumes, eggs, fruit, and sometimes milk, may have been well nourished, wealthy weanlings were fed mainly meats and bread. Even if these babies were able to digest meat—and this would have been less likely than in earlier centuries, since doctors now were railing against the custom of mothers and nurses prechewing food—on this diet they probably suffered from scurvy, rickets, bladder stones, some night blindness, and a lowered resistance to infection.

An eighteenth-century child who fussed about weaning was drugged. Laxatives, opiates, and alcohol were all used to help newly weaned children through their misery.

THE INDUSTRIAL ERA

Through most of the nineteenth century in the West, the commonly recommended age of weaning remained at about nine months, but by 1915
it had declined to seven to eight months. Several trends coincided, moreover, to make many women wean even earlier than recommended and
others fail at breastfeeding or never even attempt it. First, women spent
more time away from home; while the Industrial Revolution sent poor
women into factories, some wealthy women entered professions, and
even more joined volunteer organizations like the Women's Christian
Temperance Union and the Daughters of the American Revolution. At
the same time, the extreme prudishness of Victorian culture made public breastfeeding inconceivable, so someone besides Mother—an older
daughter in a poor family, a servant among the rich—had to stay home
and feed the baby.

Wet nurses were hired throughout the 1800s, but their popularity in
the United States gradually declined over the century. Without constant
monitoring of their diet, exercise, health, temperament, and morals,
their milk was considered hazardous to the infants in their care.
Artificial feeding therefore held hope for some women—even though until the late nineteenth century many felt "that the death warrant is
signed when the bottle is prescribed" (Apple 1987, 147).

Although ass's and goat's milk had for centuries been considered superior to cow's milk for infant feeding, cow's milk was much more widely
available. Due to mass migration to cities, however, a far smaller proportion of the population had access to pure, fresh cow's milk than in prior
centuries. In London in 1895, 80 percent of milk tested had been "sophisticated"—by removal of the cream, by dilution with water, or by the
addition of boric acid as a preservative. Chalk was often added, too, to
disguise milk that had been thinned, frequently with polluted water
(Wickes 1953). With or without the addition of water, milk delivered to
city homes was likely to have a high bacterial content. The situation was
probably little better in the United States.

Many doctors, like mothers, couldn't ignore the relationship between
artificial feeding and infant illness and death. In the nineteenth century
infant mortality rates closely paralleled the incidence of bottle feeding
among various communities, and most infant deaths were due to diarrheal infections. Because artificial foods composed of heated milk and

starch lacked vitamin C, scurvy was epidemic among infants, as was rickets.

Most doctors continued to assert the superiority of breast milk over artificial foods, but they were encountering more and more women who couldn't nurse, because of employment or disease, or, sometimes, because their adherence to doctors' feeding instructions had caused their milk to dry up. The same doctors didn't understand how they themselves might be to blame for the general decline in breastfeeding. They did recognize, however, that not all breastfed babies throve. Rickets did occur, though rarely, among breastfed children. Not until the twentieth century was it understood that the body makes vitamin D in the presence of sunlight. With their heavy clothes and love of "fair" skin, the sun-shunning Victorian rich were as prone to rickets as the urban poor, who labored in factories through the daylight hours. Breastfed babies, therefore, weren't necessarily protected from this disease. And since mixed feeding remained the norm from the early months, breastfed as well as bottle-fed babies were prone to gastrointestinal infections.

Doctors came to see breastfeeding as too demanding and difficult for most women. Certainly breast milk was the "natural food" for infants, but it was healthful only when "in proper condition," doctors believed. Pregnancy, they assumed, required weaning, as did the onset of menstruation. A baby nursed after the mother's periods resumed would supposedly suffer green stools and irritability (Wickes 1953). The child would "become delicate and puny, and every day he is nursed, will be losing instead of gaining ground" (Jefferis and Nichols 1894). Nursing after nine months, physicians thought, would cause "a tendency to brain disease," and often rickets (Jefferis and Nichols 1894). "Extreme nervousness, fright, fatigue, grief or passion" was also thought to preclude nursing (Apple 1987, 6, 110). Even a mother's nervousness about her new role, doctors believed, could cause colic, pain, constipation, and weight loss in her baby (Wickes 1953).

Breastfeeding was dangerous for women, too, physicians maintained. Nursing could cause the mother to suffer "general weariness and fatigue," "a want of refreshment from sleep," and "headaches and vertigo" (Apple 1987, 6). If she nursed beyond nine months, a mother supposedly risked deafness, blindness, and insanity (Jefferis and Nichols 1894; Verdi 1873).

Even if a mother followed all the rules, her milk was probably inadequate, doctors insisted. "The ideal breast milk is rare," wrote one (Apple

1987, 7). Beginning in the late nineteenth century, breastfed as well as bottle-fed babies were thought to require daily doses of orange or tomato juice, to prevent scurvy, and cod-liver oil, to prevent rickets. Although an initial weight loss is normal in newborns, doctors considered this unnatural, a result of overdeveloped nervous systems in civilized women. Many doctors therefore recommended supplements from the day of birth, even though some, at least, understood that this could lead to early weaning. Doctors feared, too, that a mother's milk might dry up at any time—and they reported seeing more and more of what today's writers call "insufficient milk syndrome." Physicians advised combining breast-feeding and bottle feeding throughout the nursing period to make weaning easier, when it became necessary. Their solution to dwindling milk supplies, of course, was actually the primary cause.

Doctors also promoted early weaning through their fear of overfeeding, a fear that reached a peak in the late nineteenth century. Pierre Budin, a famous French obstetrician, described overfeeding as the "scourge of infancy"; it was better to underfeed than overfeed a baby, he said, "for an underfed infant failed to gain weight but it was free from digestive troubles" (Wickes 1953). Allan Brown, a Canadian pediatrician, wrote in 1923 that overfeeding could cause not only "acute digestive disturbance" but also "the complete disappearance" of the mother's milk (Newman 1993).

For both breastfed and artificially fed infants, control was the guiding principal. "Whatever interval suits the infants is to be *strictly* enforced," said a 1925 textbook (Wickes 1953). The internationally renowned Truby King, who founded the Mothercraft Movement in New Zealand in 1907 and became an honorary member of the American Pediatric Society in 1917, insisted on feeding babies by the clock. Among his commandments were "Observe the four-hour routine to keep it holy" (Hervada and Newman 1992). Doctors forbade nursing at all during the night.

The idea that adults had to control children's natural impulses extended well beyond feeding. Truby King was as obsessed with the regularity of babies' bowel movements as with the regularity of their meals. Although King may have been extreme in his preaching, most doctors shared his basic philosophy. Not only was a mother not to give her baby the breast when the baby cried at an unappointed time, they believed, she was not even to pick the baby up. Dr. Frederick Rossiter (1908) agreed: Picking up or nursing a crying baby would "cultivate self-indulgence and a lack of self-control. . . . Because of neglect to train their children properly, a large proportion of parents are slaves to their children, and are ruled instead of ruling." Children, like all of nature, had to be disciplined, regulated, tamed.

> "How often do we see the young infant stop crying at two weeks when it is picked up by either parent? Herein lies the potential juvenile court case. Unless the parents are guided by the physician even at this early stage, the infant soon learns to put one over on its parents."
>
> ALLAN BROWN, 1923 (NEWMAN 1993)

Fortunately, doctors had only moderate influence in nineteenth-century America. Until the late eighteenth century, doctors were few in this country, and those doctors in practice had been educated in Europe. Throughout the next century the profession generally had low status. This was for good reason; according to Richard and Dorothy Wertz, authors of *Lying In* (1979, 51), "throughout much of the nineteenth century a doctor could obtain a diploma and begin practice with as little as four months' attendance at a school that might have no laboratories, no dissections, and no clinical training." Even in 1910, 90 percent of doctors had no college education, and most doctors had attended small, proprietary, short-lived, and substandard medical schools (Wertz and Wertz 1979, 55). Doctors were gradually able to build a clientele, however, by getting a share in, and finally taking over, the midwifery business. Although until after 1900 immigrant women continued to prefer their midwives, Victorian culture found midwifery unsuitable for women. Middle- and upper-class mothers therefore happily turned to doctors to attend them in childbirth.

In the latter half of the nineteenth century, physicians found another way to expand their practices. Sometimes genuinely alarmed at the high rate of infant mortality and its apparent association with artificial feeding, doctors found they could profit by becoming authorities on artificial infant foods. They debated the relative merits of fresh and heated cow's milk, they devised formulas for laboratory or home modification of milk, and they analyzed and evaluated the new but quickly proliferating commercial infant foods.

The chemists, pharmacists, and businessmen who devised and marketed these artificial foods often began with benevolent motives. The first of these men was Justus von Liebig, a German chemist who in the 1860s created "the most perfect substitute for Mother's milk," as one advertisement described it. Composed of cow's milk with wheat and malt flours, Liebig's Food was sold in the United States from 1869 on, and became a model for other manufacturers to follow. Gustav Mellin, an English chemist who followed Liebig's theories, devised a similar product that was easier to prepare, by diluting the mixture in plain milk and water. Henri Nestle, a Swiss merchant, created a mixture of "good Swiss milk," sugar, and flour cooked with malt, to which only water had to be added. About the same time, Gail Borden devised a way of preserving milk by adding sugar; his Eagle Brand milk was sold for both infants and general home use. James Horlick, a pharmacist who had worked for Mellin in England before immigrating to the United States, combined dry milk and malt flour in Horlick's Malted Milk, which was advertised as a food for infants and invalids. These products were among many artificial infant foods that were widely advertised and sold in the United States from the late 1860s through the 1890s.

While many doctors experimented with artificial infant foods and praised them, others were more critical. No formula could be truly "complete," some rightly believed, without the addition of raw milk or some other supplement that would prevent scurvy. Most doctors also maintained that different babies needed different formulas, and that each baby needed changing formulas as he or she grew. The diet of every infant therefore needed a doctor's oversight. Doctors prescribed formulas for mothers to prepare at home; they set up milk laboratories, where formulas could be prepared for home delivery, and milk stations, which were dairies and milk laboratories combined; and they invented devices for sterilizing and pasteurizing milk at home. One doctor invented the rubber bottle nipple, in 1884, and others improved upon it.

Doctors couldn't control all artificial infant feeding, however, as long as commercial infant foods were advertised and sold, with mixing instructions, directly to the public. The American Medical Association therefore began offering its seal of approval only to infant food manufacturers who published ads solely in medical journals—not in women's magazines—and provided feeding instructions solely to doctors. The manufacturers complied; they started marketing formulas as nonprescription but "ethical" products, whose use was difficult without a doctor's direction. (Only in the late twentieth century did formula makers resume printing feeding instructions on their packages.) Doctors "increasingly insisted that mothers go to private physicians or well-baby clinics for advice on child care in general and infant feeding in particular" (Apple 1987, 86).

The doctors' practice of changing infant formulas kept mothers and babies coming back. As a result, "manipulating the composition of formulas heralded the advent of pediatrics as a specialty" (Newman 1993). Not only pediatricians benefited from artificial feeding, however; by the late 1920s at least 25 percent of general practitioners' cases consisted in directing artificial infant feeding.

Certain cultural trends at the turn of the twentieth century made middle- and upper-class women particularly susceptible to doctors' advice. Science became equated with progress. Housewives came to see themselves as domestic scientists, who studied, measured, and engineered their way through their cooking, cleaning, and child-rearing duties. At the same time, doctors overcame their profession's poor reputation by identifying medicine with science. They promoted themselves as scientific experts who would replace the traditional knowledge of "old women" and "uneducated nurses."

In the late 1800s, child-care books and pamphlets, women's magazines, and domestic-science classes began leading women to believe that maternal instinct was useless and even dangerous. "Maternal instinct left alone," wrote "a trained mother" in *Good Housekeeping* in 1911, "succeeds in killing a large proportion of the babies born into this world" (Apple 1987, 101). Much more valuable than instinct in the work of raising children was scientific instruction. Since most mothers couldn't acquire a physician's education, however, proponents of scientific motherhood gradually came to believe that mothers needed expert advice more than formal instruction. More and more, these writers accorded physicians the major role in making decisions about infant feeding. On this subject, advised a 1935 mothering manual, "the doctor should decide—you must rely on his advice completely; he must lay down the laws you are to follow out and you are to ask no one else about them" (Apple 1987, 130).

Physicians' frequent and dire warnings about prolonged breastfeeding indicate that nursing into the second year was probably common in the nineteenth century. By 1915, however, all but 3 percent of U.S. mothers weaned by the baby's thirteenth month (Whitehead 1985). Still, most mothers breastfed successfully, at least through the early months, until hospital birth became popular. More than any other influence, probably, the transition from home birth to hospital birth doomed women to lactation failure and early weaning. In the nineteenth century, maternity hospitals were asylums for poor, homeless, or unmarried urban women. Wealthier women avoided these hospitals, where childbed fever was often epidemic. But in the 1880s obstetricians improved their sanitary practices, developed new medical skills, and cleaned up their image. Women came to see hospitals as safe, clean, and comfortable places to give birth and to rest for two to three weeks afterward.

In the 1920s, maternity hospitals began to offer another attraction: "twilight sleep," or drugged, painless birth. Most women loved the idea. Whereas in 1900 fewer than 5 percent of U.S. women delivered in hospitals, in 1939 50 percent did, many of them enabled to do so by the automobile. In 1950, over 80 percent of U.S. women delivered their babies in hospitals (Wertz and Wertz 1979, 48, 133, 135).

Hospital routines made it hard for a woman to establish lactation. Babies were separated from their mothers right after birth and cared for in big nurseries by nurses wearing face masks to prevent the spread of germs. Since the mother's germs were considered just as dangerous to the baby as the nurses' were, hospitals instituted feeding routines like this one, described in a journal for hospital administrators:

> The breast is cleansed thoroughly each day with soap and water. Before the baby is brought to the mother, her hands are carefully washed with soap and water, and she is warned to touch nothing after that until her baby is at the breast. The binder is unpinned, with the mother resting on her side. The nurse, with scrubbed hands, lays a sterile receiver by the mother and the child is placed upon that. After the nursing, the nipple and aureola are sponged with 35 per cent alcohol, and a fresh sterile binder is applied (Apple 1987, 120).

Made to feel dirty and helpless by these routines, women often gave up breastfeeding because they believed their milk was "bad."

Feedings were usually every four hours, sometimes every eight. Whether a baby cried between feedings, or slept during them, didn't matter. Each nursing was followed by a bottle feeding. By limiting nursings, hospital routines often delayed or limited women's milk production. After "bad" milk, the cause most often cited for giving up breastfeeding was lack of milk.

As hospital births became more common and physicians' influence grew, both physicians and mothers came to see artificial feeding as normal. As early as the 1880s, some doctors preferred artificial feeding to breastfeeding because "it is easier to control cows than women," and because with bottles a doctor could be sure how much a baby was getting (Apple 1987, 56). Colic, doctors thought, was harder to cure in breastfed babies, since it was due to the mother's nervousness. And since medical schools provided no training in solving breastfeeding difficulties, the only solution most doctors could offer to such difficulties was the bottle.

Although women's magazines, home-economics textbooks, home medical manuals, and booklets distributed by infant food manufacturers all asserted that breastfeeding was natural and best, they had nothing else to say about breastfeeding except that many women couldn't do it. Bottle feeding was considered inevitable at some point in every baby's life. "Even if you are breast-feeding," advised *Parents' Magazine* (Apple 1987, 126), "you may be ordered by your doctor to give supplementary feedings by bottle; so it is fairly safe to count on bottles and their attendant equipment."

> "A good breast is a blessing, a poor one may be a 'delusion, a mockery, and a snare.'"
>
> FROM AN ARTICLE IN *BABYHOOD*, 1902 (APPLE 1987, 109)

Throughout most of the twentieth century, women increasingly declined to breastfeed at all, or weaned to the bottle within a few months after giving birth. Between 1910 and 1920, 82 to 92 percent of U.S. one-month-olds were exclusively breastfed, yet by 1948, 35 percent of hospital-born babies were weaned at discharge; another 27 percent were receiving formula as well as breast milk. In 1958, 63 percent of babies were weaned at discharge, and 16 percent were getting both breast- and bottle feedings. The early 1970s marked the low point in breastfeeding in the United States: Fewer than 25 percent of babies were receiving breast milk at discharge, and all but 8 percent were weaned by three to four months of age.

Not only did babies of nonnursing mothers receive cow's milk- or soy-based formula instead of breast milk, but they were also fed cereals and strained fruits and vegetables from a very early age. Throughout the 1950s and 1960s, most U.S. babies were fed commercially prepared semi-solid foods before they were even able to hold their heads up, much less digest these foods well. By the early 1970s, most babies received such foods by the age of six weeks, and many were fed them within a day or two of birth.

In the mid-twentieth century, according to Whiting and Child (1953), U.S. weaning practices, though severe, were not among the world's harshest. But the reason most U.S. women felt no need to apply foul substances to their breasts or slap their children away was that these children were weaned while still helpless infants. Of 52 societies Whiting and Child studied, the initial deprivation of the child's oral interests was greater in the U. S. middle class than in all but one other society.

In the latter half of the 1970s, to the surprise of many people, breastfeeding regained popularity in Western countries. By 1980 more than half of U.S. women who gave birth in hospitals nursed their babies. In 1985 60 percent did, and 35 percent were still breastfeeding at four months after birth. A small but determined minority of women were nursing for one year, two years, three years, or even longer.

What forces brought about this reversal? Beginning in the 1940s, a few hospitals initiated the policy of "rooming in," by which a mother was allowed to keep her baby with her for all or part of the day, and thereby learn to nurse her baby without the interference of nurses and their bottles. By 1980 rooming in was common in U.S. hospitals. A good deal of credit, too, must go to La Leche League, a grassroots organization founded in 1956 to promote breastfeeding and "natural" mothering through mother-to-mother discussion. Broad cultural changes, however, may have done most to foster the new trend. In the wake of the turbulent 1960s and early 1970s, breastfeeding resurged along with interest in natural foods, alternative medicine, and non-Western cultures. Young adults of the middle and upper classes, fearing that all of Western society was on a racetrack to self-destruction, dug in their heels. Women struggled against hospital routines, physicians' advice, and relatives' opinions for the right to nurse their babies. They stopped scheduling feedings and forcing solid foods into babies too young to digest them; some began to breastfeed in public; and some let their children go on nursing for months or years after doctors or relatives said they should quit. These women were leading a shift in Western child-rearing practices toward those generally characteristic of the rest of humankind.

NURSING AND WEANING TODAY

After the mid-1980s, as more women entered the work force, the U.S. breastfeeding rate decreased somewhat. Wealthier, more educated, and older women were far more likely to breastfeed than others, and to wean later. Poor and immigrant women tended to prefer artificial feeding. In part, this was due to the government-sponsored Supplemental Food Program for Women, Infants, and Children (WIC), which inadvertently encouraged bottle feeding by displaying and giving away huge quantities of infant formula. In 1985, 29 percent of U.S. infants were enrolled in WIC, and the percentage of them who were breastfed was only about half that of other babies.

By 1990, however, breastfeeding rates began to increase again, even though more and more women were going back to work before their children's first birthdays. Women who worked full time were now as likely as unemployed women to start out breastfeeding, although they tended to wean earlier. Many women dropped their work hours to part time so that they could continue nursing longer.

The support of scientists and public health organizations encouraged women to start and continue breastfeeding. In 1989, an ever-growing body of research documenting the benefits of breast milk and the dangers of early supplementation provoked U.S. Surgeon General C. Everett Koop to publicly encourage breastfeeding. In 1991 the World Health Organization issued a declaration in support of breastfeeding, and in the early 1990s WIC began providing advice, extra food, and even breast pumps for its nursing clients. The American Academy of Pediatrics formed its Task Force on Breastfeeding in 1994, and in 2002 the Academy began recommending that infants be offered only breast milk for the first six months after birth, and that breastfeeding continue throughout the first year and then as long as mother and baby desire.

Other probable causes for the resurgence of breastfeeding include improvements in maternity care, breast pumps, and workplace rights for nursing women, and the growing numbers of professional lactation consultants and of female physicians. Many studies have shown social support to be the most important factor in determining whether women start and continue breastfeeding. As more and more women can look to their own mothers, as well as peers and professionals, as breastfeeding models, we can expect the breastfeeding rates to continue their rise.

In 2004, over 70 percent of U.S. mothers of newborns were breastfeeding. Thirty-six percent were still nursing at six months, and almost 18 percent were nursing at twelve months. Only one ethnic group, non-Hispanic African Americans, breastfed at a low rate, just over 50 percent. Still, this represents a tremendous increase over 1989, when only 23 percent of black women nursed their babies. Breastfeeding rates also increased substantially among young women, poor women, and high-school dropouts.

Healthy People 2010, a national initiative to improve the health of all Americans, aims by the year 2010 to have 75 percent of U.S. mothers starting out breastfeeding, 50 percent breastfeeding when their babies are six months old, and 25 percent still nursing at the end of the first year. Fourteen states have met the first goal, but only two, Oregon and Utah, have met the last two. As a nation, we have a long way to go. Three months after giving birth, over half of American women who started out breastfeeding have begun feeding their babies formula. Just as in Victorian times, early artificial feeding is leading to early weaning.

THE HAZARDS OF FORMULA FEEDING

Today most women who wean in the first year switch to feeding commercial infant formula, a mixture of cow's milk or soybean products and various other substances. Is formula feeding really all that bad? Today's formulas, actually, are probably the best artificial infant foods ever devised. But they are not the same as breast milk. Although most doctors avoid saying so, out of fear of alienating some clients, formula-fed babies are generally less healthy than breastfed babies. On average, the cognitive development of formula-fed infants is slightly inferior. Breast milk protects against disease and promotes optimal brain growth. Formula does neither of these things.

Compared with breast milk, infant formulas are deficient in many essential nutrients and oversupplied with others. Great debate surrounds the topic of what ingredients should go into formula, and formula manufacturers are constantly challenged to improve their formulations as more is learned about the composition of human milk. Every year, formula makers change their recipes because of new evidence that another substance or nutrient in breast milk is important for optimal infant growth and development. As Dr. Derrick Jelliffe explained, "Hindsight shows the story of formula production to be a succession of errors. Each stumble is dealt with and heralded as yet another breakthrough, leading to further imbalances and then more modifications" (*Wall Street Journal,* March 20, 1980). Some critics have said that the mass feeding of artificial human milk is one of the most extensive experiments ever undertaken on human beings.

No matter how hard manufacturers struggle to reproduce human milk, they can't do it. Breast milk is alive with the mother's antibodies, living cells that fight off bacteria and viruses. A breastfed infant takes in about 100 million live cells per day, many of which survive 48 hours or longer. An infant needs her mother's antibodies because her own immune system is very immature and poorly equipped to fight infection on its own. Even at one year of age, a baby's immune system functions at only about 60 percent of the adult level.

Formula, which has no live antibodies, is strongly associated with high rates of infection. Ear infections occur as many as four times more often in formula-fed than in breastfed infants (Saarinen 1982; Duncan et al. 1993; Aniansson et al. 1994). Besides being painful, repeated ear infections cause language difficulties, which are evidenced by lower reading comprehension and more need for speech therapy and remedial teaching (Luotonen et al. 1996; Teele et al. 1990; Schilder et al. 1993).

Formula-fed babies suffer more infections of other kinds, too. Respiratory infections, including colds, bronchitis, and pneumonia, are twice as likely in formula-fed babies (Wright et al. 1989). Diarrheal infections occur three to five times more often in the formula-fed infant (Feachem and Koblinsky 1984; Popkin et al. 1990; Scariati et al. 1997). Urinary tract infections and meningitis, a life-threatening infection of the lining of the brain and spinal cord, are also more common among formula-fed babies (Pisacane et al. 1992; Cochi et al. 1986). In fact, a formula-fed baby in the United States is ten times more likely to be hospitalized for a serious infection than a breastfed baby is (Fallot et al. 1980).

Formula feeding is associated with vulnerability not only to acute infections but to other illnesses as well. Formula-fed babies are more likely to become overweight later in life, and obesity is associated with many diseases (Harder et al. 2005). Formula feeding may be responsible for up to a quarter of all cases of Type I (insulin-dependent) diabetes (Mayer et al. 1988; Scariati et al. 1997). Children breastfed less than six months or not at all have a higher risk of developing childhood leukemia, and their risk of developing lymphoma, or cancer of the glands, is five to eight times higher than that of children nursed more than six months (Davis et al. 1988; Shu et al. 1995). Pyloric stenosis, an obstruction of the stomach that requires surgical repair, is more common among formula-fed infants (Habbick et al. 1989). Formula feeding has also been linked with chronic intestinal disorders such as celiac disease, ulcerative colitis, and Crohn's disease (Greco et al. 1988; Koletzko et al. 1989; Ivarsson et al. 2002). And formula feeding is thought to interfere with infants' immune response to vaccinations, so they aren't protected from infection as long as breastfed children are (Hahn-Zoric et al. 1990).

According to the National Institute of Environmental Health Sciences, four infants out of every thousand born in the United States die because they do not receive their mother's milk. Each year 500 U.S. infants and young children die from diarrhea, an illness usually associated with formula feeding (Ho et al. 1988). Besides protecting against life-threatening diarrheal and respiratory illness, breastfeeding protects against fatal types of infant botulism, which may cause Sudden Infant Death Syndrome, or SIDS (Arnon 1986). SIDS occurs much more frequently among formula-fed babies than among breastfed babies (Mitchell et al. 1991; Ford et al. 1993). One large study determined that for each month of exclusive breastfeeding, the SIDS rate was reduced by 50 percent (Frederickson et al. 1993).

Unlike formula, breast milk promotes the growth and development of the human brain and nervous system. Numerous studies confirm that young children who have been formula-fed generally have lower intellectual ability than those who have been breastfed (Morley et al. 1988;

Morrow-Tlucak et al. 1988; Bauer et al. 1991; Taylor and Wadsworth 1984; Lucas et al. 1992). The longer a child is breastfed, in fact, the higher her I.Q. is likely to be. Formula-fed children earn lower scores on standardized reading, language, and math tests, as well as I.Q. tests, than do children who have been breastfed (Fergusson et al. 1982). The cognitive benefits of breast milk persist into young adulthood, when former breastfed babies show higher performance on standardized tests of reading, math, and general scholastic ability (Horwood and Fergusson 1998). And formula feeding is associated with speech disorders, particularly in boys, with learning disabilities, and with infantile autism (Broad and Duganzich 1983; Dorner and Grychtolik 1978; Collipp et al. 1983; Tanoue and Oda 1989).

Formula-fed babies are more likely to suffer from allergies than are breastfed babies. Many infants are allergic to cow's milk formula (Jakobsson and Lindberg 1978), and as many as half of these babies are also allergic to soy formula. These allergies may contribute to the development of others. Formula-fed babies, particularly those born into families with allergies, suffer more allergy-induced wheezing, diarrhea, and vomiting than do babies who are breastfed (Merrett et al. 1988; Wright et al. 1995). Because allergies inflame breathing passages, formula-fed babies also tend to have prolonged colds.

Some formulas have been found to be toxic, because of either normal manufacturing processes or gross manufacturing errors. Most formulas contain contaminants such as aluminum and iodine; some also contain bacteria. Researchers worry about how the high levels of iodine in formula may affect infants' thyroid function (Fisher 1989). They also wonder about the possible effects of some formulas' very high aluminum levels—up to 20 times higher than that of breast milk (Bishop et al. 1989). Bacterial contamination of formula, which has occurred from time to time, has made babies sick (Simmons et al. 1989). Powdered forms of formula are especially liable to be contaminated, since, unlike ready-to-feed formulas or liquid concentrates, they cannot be sterilized by the manufacturer without damage to the ingredients. As many as 35 percent of powdered formulas are contaminated with *Enterobacter sakazakii,* a pathogen linked to blood infections, serious gut infections, and meningitis (Kandhai et al. 2004). Newborns and infants born at low birth weights who become ill with *E. sakazakii* have mortality rates as high as 80 percent.

Potential hazards exist in the preparation of bottles, too. Because an estimated 20 percent of U.S. homes have tap water that is contaminated with lead, feeding powdered formula or formula concentrate combined with tap water can lead to lead poisoning in the baby. Lead poisoning can cause permanent damage to the brain, nervous system, kidneys, and red blood cells. Lead may also be a cause of dental cavities. Boiling tap water to prepare sterile formula for feeding can increase the lead levels even more (Shannon and Graf 1992).

Formula presents more hazards when it isn't mixed precisely. Overdiluting formula with water can stunt a baby's growth. Underdiluting formula can tax a baby's kidneys and digestive system, and can lead to dehydration. Formulas mixed by parents are often over- or underdiluted (McJunkin et al. 1987).

The use of bottles in formula feeding presents other dangers for babies. Bottle feeding can cause an orthodontic disorder, the improper meeting of the upper and lower teeth (Labbok and Hendershot 1987). The common practice of microwaving bottles not only can lead to burns in the mouth but can also destroy vitamins in the formula. Bottle propping, another common practice, can result in choking. Infants allowed to feed themselves also experience less of the touching and social interaction that all babies need.

Formula is expensive. In the United States, a year's worth of formula concentrate for one baby costs $1,200 to $2,800, and a year's worth of ready-to-feed formula costs $1,200 to $4,000. To save money, parents often switch to plain cow's milk before their babies turn a year old. Cow's milk, whether whole, low-fat, or non-fat, is a poor food for a baby. Since cow's milk contains little iron, feeding it in place of breast milk or formula can lead to iron-deficiency anemia, the most common nutritional problem in U.S. infants. Iron deficiency has been associated with subtle behavioral differences that cannot be corrected with later iron supplementation (Lozoff et al. 1987). Feeding cow's milk can also lead to intestinal blood loss in some babies (Ziegler et al. 1990). The levels of protein and sodium in cow's milk are too high for babies, and the levels of vitamin C, vitamin E, and copper are too low.

Not only are formula-fed babies at increased risk for various illnesses, but so are their mothers. Women who breastfeed for two years or longer lower their risk of developing breast cancer by as much as 50 percent (Layde et al. 1989; Zheng et al. 2000). Breastfeeding also protects against ovarian cancer (Gwinn et al. 1990), against osteoporosis (Aloia et al. 1985; Koetting and Wardlaw 1988), and possibly against cervical cancer (Brock et al. 1989).

Mothers who do not breastfeed may get pregnant again before they are physically or emotionally ready. Whereas women who forego breast-feeding become fertile only four to six weeks after delivery, women who are exclusively breastfeeding and have not resumed their periods have 98 percent protection from another pregnancy for the first six months after birth without using other birth control methods (Kennedy et al. 1989).

Feeding methods affect a woman's adjustment to her role as a mother. The hormones produced in breastfeeding stimulate feelings of affection and relaxation, and these feelings enhance nurturing behavior. The necessity of physical contact in breastfeeding probably also makes a mother more attentive.

Although researchers have done little investigation on how feeding methods affect a woman's sense of self, every mother can testify on this matter. Women who for one reason or another were convinced that they couldn't nurse talk about the pain, regret, and grief that failed breast-feeding evokes even years later. Women who have breastfed successfully, in contrast, testify to a rewarding experience in which they typically take great pride.

Infant formula is not inherently evil; it can be a great convenience when mother and child must be separated, and it provides the best nutrition possible for a baby when breast milk simply isn't available. In the next two chapters we'll tell you how to go about weaning a baby to formula as safely as possible. But to rely on formula unnecessarily would be foolish. Even in the twenty-first century, too many women wean early because of shame about their bodies, ignorance of how breastfeeding works, and distrust of children's ability to know and express their true needs. If we can sort out our feelings about nursing and understand their social roots, if we seek out teachers with practical experience, and if we trust ourselves and our children as the best teachers of all, we can often overcome the practical difficulties that may lead to weaning long before a child is physically or emotionally ready.

two

WEANING BEFORE
FOUR MONTHS

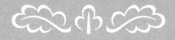

Y OU MAY BE CONSIDERING WEANING your young baby for any number of reasons. Like many new mothers, you may feel unsupported in your efforts to breastfeed, alone among your friends, or let down by your mate, by your family, by your baby's doctor, or by your own doctor. Perhaps you are facing a return to work or some other separation from your baby. Or maybe breastfeeding has not been what you expected, and you think weaning will make things better.

Whatever your situation, it is important to consider your circumstances thoroughly and measure the hardships you face against the value of breastfeeding to you and, most importantly, to your baby. Read, or review, "The Hazards of Formula Feeding" in Chapter 1. Although weaning a young baby to a bottle is relatively quick and easy, it can be difficult to reverse.

Nursing Your Young Baby

Before you gave birth, you may have assumed that you would nurse your baby. Or, perhaps, like many women, you chose breastfeeding after much consideration because of the health advantages it offers a baby and the close mother-child relationship it fosters. In either case, you were committed to providing your baby with the very best start. But before having a baby you could hardly anticipate the incredible changes that would occur after birth—in your body, your role, your feelings, your relationships, and your energy level. Nor could you know what sort of temperament your baby would have, or anticipate the round-the-clock realities of child care and breastfeeding.

Perhaps you were led to believe that breastfeeding is entirely instinctive and easy. Yet the truth is that it can sometimes be difficult, especially during the early weeks. Although breastfeeding is a natural consequence to giving birth, it does not always come naturally; it is a learned skill that usually takes a mother and baby several weeks to master. Sometimes they need an experienced person to help. Maybe you turned to your doctor for assistance with breastfeeding, and went away unsatisfied. Most doctors simply don't have the time or the skill necessary to help women overcome breastfeeding complications and obstacles.

Human infants are meant to be nursed frequently and without restriction. Whereas some species have mammary structures designed to be emptied only twice a day, a woman's breast, which produces milk continuously, must be emptied often to maintain production. The more your breast is drained, the more milk it will produce. If you nurse your baby infrequently, your milk production will decrease and ultimately you may not be able to meet his growth needs.

Babies nurse frequently because breast milk, with its low protein content, is so quickly digested. With frequent nursing, human milk provides an almost continuous supply of nutrients essential for brain growth. Cow's milk, in contrast, promotes rapid bone and muscle growth, not rapid brain growth, and, with its high protein content, it requires less frequent feedings.

The composition of human milk also promotes frequent contact between mother and baby. Whereas some species hide their babies away and go off grazing or searching for food, our closest relatives, other primates, carry their babies along everywhere until the babies are old enough to follow close behind. In their first months, human infants are even more helpless than other primate young. The frequent contact that breastfeeding requires provides not only physical protection but the social stimulation essential to infant development. Close physical contact also helps develop the sense of trust that babies need to survive in the world.

Still, having your baby with you at all times and nursing him whenever he seems hungry may seem impractical in today's world. Although breastfeeding is generally considered to be the ideal infant feeding method, it is not supported in public or in the workplace, where a woman may spend much of her time. Yet many women successfully fit breastfeeding into their lives by acknowledging the needs of their babies and the demands of nursing them, and by managing their other commitments and activities without sacrificing breastfeeding.

During the early weeks of breastfeeding, mothers typically experience an array of emotions and feelings about breastfeeding. You may be feeling the highest highs and the lowest lows you've ever known. You may be struggling with latch-on problems, with soreness, or with establishing an adequate milk supply. Trying to interpret your baby's crying and his feeding and sleep patterns (or adapt to the lack of any such patterns) may consume most of your time and energy. Certainly, it is during these early weeks that mothers tend to react most negatively to nursing. In fact, half of all women who start out nursing give it up during the first six weeks after birth. They are prompted to wean by some difficulty or other, which may be compounded by unrealistic expectations of motherhood and breastfeeding.

After the first several weeks, you may have other reasons to consider weaning, such as the difficulties of managing occasional separations from your baby, returning to work, or reviving your appearance, marriage, or sex life. Whatever phase of nursing you're in, if you're struggling with a problem you may find it hard to imagine that things will get better. Resolving the problem can seem to take an eternity. For most nursing mothers, though, things usually do get better. Most concerns can be eased with good information, support, and practical planning.

You may go through phases of loving breastfeeding and of hating it, but most of the time your feelings are probably mixed. Even the happiest nursing mother sometimes feels ambivalent about nursing—and about other parental responsibilities as well. Throughout your parenting years, the wants and needs of your child will undoubtedly collide with your own desires from time to time. Ambivalent feelings do not necessarily mean you should stop what you're doing and try something radically new. However long you nurse, it helps to appreciate that breastfeeding, like mothering in general, just has its ups and downs.

In solving breastfeeding problems, having support is important. Ideally, you should have unwavering support from your mate, your family, your friends, and your health-care providers; in reality, you might not get support from any of them. Fortunately, there are people in almost every community to whom a mother can turn when breastfeeding difficulties arise. You may feel reluctant to reach out for help; Kathleen often talks with women who have struggled for days or even weeks before calling her breastfeeding hotline, and some even apologize for "bothering" her. Don't struggle alone! To locate sources of help, see the Appendix.

Possible Reasons to Wean Your Young Baby

UNRESOLVED BREASTFEEDING DIFFICULTIES

If you have been struggling with some breastfeeding difficulty, weaning and formula feeding may seem to be the best solution. But if you're not sure that early weaning is necessary, the discussion and suggestions that follow may help you continue breastfeeding.

Sore Nipples

Tender nipples are a common complaint during the first few days of nursing. Some women, though, suffer from extremely sore nipples when they first start breastfeeding, or they continue to experience pain while feeding long past the early days. Others get sore nipples after a period of comfortable nursing. In any case, sore nipples can make what should be a pleasurable experience a dreaded chore.

Perhaps you have already tried various remedies for nipple pain suggested by friends or health professionals. Sore nipples are usually the result of one of three things: poor positioning of the baby on the breast, faulty sucking, or an underlying skin condition on the nipples. Sore nipples are not normal, and they certainly can be remedied.

Cracked Nipples Due to Faulty Attachment. Some women develop painful, cracked nipples during the first few days of nursing. This typically happens because the newborn is poorly latched on to the breast during feedings. Painful cracking of the nipples can be caused by an infection (see "Irritated or Burning Nipples," pages 30–32), but when this problem occurs during the first few days of nursing the usual reason is that the newborn is poorly latched on to the breast during feedings. If you have had sore nipples since you started nursing, review the description of positioning and attachment techniques in the Appendix.

If the nipple pain is very intense, you may want to stop breastfeeding temporarily, and rent a fully automatic electric breast pump to express the milk for your baby while your nipples heal. A fully automatic pump will probably be gentler on a cracked nipple than your baby is, and the pump will help you maintain your milk supply.

A fully automatic breast pump is the most comfortable, efficient, and easy-to-use kind, and it works better than other pumps in maintaining the milk supply. When you rent or buy a fully automatic pump, you can also buy a double-collection kit, which allows for pumping both breasts at once, for a total of only about ten to twelve minutes. Long-term rental of a fully automatic pump costs only one-third to one-half the cost of formula for the same period; buying one costs about as much as two to three months' worth of formula. See the Appendix for help in locating a pump.

After a few days of pumping, you may be ready to start nursing again. (Be sure to review the description of correct positioning, in the Appendix, to minimize the possibility of the soreness recurring.) Resume breastfeeding slowly. Nurse twice a day at first, while continuing to pump for other feedings. Then slowly increase the number of daily feedings, paying careful attention to your latch-on technique, until you are back to full-time nursing.

If after a few days of pumping your nipples don't seem to be healing, consider discussing the situation with your primary-care doctor, a lactation professional, or even a dermatologist. Cracked nipples are often infected with bacteria. The infection typically delays healing and often leads to mastitis. A prescribed oral antibiotic may speed healing.

Once your nipples have healed and you are beginning to breastfeed again, nursing shouldn't hurt. If it does, find out why; the most likely cause is an incorrect attachment of the baby on your breast. Besides reviewing the description of correct positioning, in the Appendix, you might consider having a lactation professional observe you and your baby during a feeding. (You can find a lactation professional by calling one of the numbers listed in the Appendix.)

> If you must stop nursing temporarily, use an automatic pump every two to three hours during the day and evening, and whenever the baby wakes for a feeding at night. If only one breast is affected, pump that side while continuing to nurse on the other breast. You will probably need to give the baby some or all of the expressed milk.

Faulty Sucking. Occasionally a mother develops sore or injured nipples because her baby has a faulty suck. This happens, for example, when a baby is "tongue-tied"; that is, when the frenulum, a string-like tissue under the tongue, is attached too close to the tip of the tongue. This condition prevents the tongue from extending much past the gums, and it can lead to a "biting" or "pinching" sensation during feedings. Clipping the frenulum is simple, quick, and bloodless or nearly so; your baby's doctor or a dentist can do this during an office visit. A lactation professional can be helpful in identifying a frenulum in need of clipping or any other sucking difficulties.

Irritated or Burning Nipples. Some mothers say that their nipples sting or burn during feedings. There isn't much professional literature on this kind of soreness because it is less common than other kinds, but it can be very frustrating for a nursing mother. If your nipples are irritated, they may look slightly red. Careful positioning of the baby for nursing, and other measures such as air-drying the nipples, may do little to ease the pain. Try talking to a doctor, preferably a dermatologist. Many mothers with longstanding soreness of this type get rapid relief from a moderate- or high-strength anti-inflammatory ointment, sometimes in combination with an antibiotic ointment. A California dermatologist has identified a variety of skin conditions on the nipples, including various forms of dermatitis, eczema, and impetigo.

One cause of nipple burning and irritation is yeast. A yeast infection on the nipples, which often occurs after a period of comfortable nursing, may make the nipples appear redder than normal and sometimes wet and "soggy" looking. The nipples can even develop painful cracks. The areola, the dark area surrounding the nipple, may peel or break out in a red, dotty rash. Some mothers also complain of burning or stabbing pains in their breasts. This infection occurs when a baby with thrush—a yeast infection in the mouth—transfers the infection to her mother's nipples. A doctor may diagnose thrush in a baby but say nothing about the mother's nipples, which should be treated at the same time as the oral infection.

Unless you already know that your baby has thrush, carefully inspect your baby's mouth. You may see small white patches, or "curds," inside her lips, inside her cheeks, and sometimes on her tongue; the patches will not easily rub off. Some yeast infections don't show up in the baby's mouth, but are evidenced by a diaper rash; this is more likely after four months of age, when a baby's immune system is more mature. A yeast diaper rash is seen most often on and around the penis or labia; it often resembles a mild burn; it may peel; and it does not respond to ordinary remedies for diaper rash. Sometimes the rash appears as just a patch of red dots. Typically babies with yeast infections have a lot of gas, and they may be fussy.

If the nipple pain is very intense, you might want to stop breastfeeding temporarily, and rent a fully automatic electric breast pump (see page 185) to express milk for your baby until the yeast can be treated and your nipples improve.

Yeast infections require regular and thorough treatment of both mother and baby to prevent recurrence. The usual treatment is 1 milliliter of nystatin suspension, placed by dropper in the baby's mouth after every other nursing, or four times daily, for fourteen days. Nystatin is most effective when given right after a feeding, so that it isn't washed out of the baby's mouth by nursing or bottle feeding. Drop half of the dose into each side of your baby's mouth; she should swallow most of the medicine. You can swab some more into the affected areas with a cotton-tipped applicator. For your nipples, use nystatin cream or some other antifungal medication; your baby's medicine can be used instead, but it might prove to be less effective. Apply the cream to your nipples at least after every other nursing or pumping. The same cream can also help clear any diaper rash. Nystatin in either form must be prescribed by a physician, but Lotrimin AF, Micatin, and Monistat 7—any of which can be used on your nipples and on your baby's diaper rash—are available over the counter.

Many women with thrush-infected nipples find nystatin suspension less than fully effective in treating oral thrush. This may be because the drug does not remain in the baby's mouth long enough. Another medicine you could try, along with nystatin suspension or separately, is 1 percent solution of gentian violet, which you can purchase in a drugstore without a prescription. Once or twice a day for three days, put two drops of gentian violet on a cotton-tipped swab, and thoroughly swab the parts of the baby's mouth where you can see thrush. The solution will temporarily stain the baby's mouth purple; take care in applying it so that you don't stain anything else. Turn your baby onto her stomach for a few minutes after you've swabbed her mouth, to minimize the amount she swallows. (Although gentian violet is very effective in ridding the mouth of yeast, when it is used more often than twice a day, or longer than three days in a row, it can cause ulcers in a baby's mouth. If the thrush isn't gone after a three-day course, wait several days before trying again.)

Also important when treating a yeast infection are these measures:

◆ Change your nursing pads at each feeding.

◆ Boil daily for five minutes pacifiers, bottle nipples, and any breast pump parts that come in contact with your breast or milk.

◆ Replace weekly all artificial nipples, including pacifiers.

Some mothers experience burning nipples even after their babies' thrush is gone—although the soreness may have lessened somewhat, the irritation continues. This may be due to the preservatives used in some of the generic nystatin creams. A dermatologist can help determine whether the yeast is cleared up and can prescribe medication to stop the nipple irritation.

Plugged Nipple Pore. A plugged nipple opening is another possible cause of nipple pain. Some women with plugged nipple pores also complain of breast pain, and sometimes an area in the breast may not empty with nursing. The nipple in these cases looks normal in color except for a white spot on the tip, which is particularly visible right after the baby comes off the breast. See "Plugged Ducts," page 49, for further information.

Difficult Latch-on and Refusal to Nurse

A baby who is not latching on and is unable to breastfeed presents a frustrating situation. Occasionally a baby is born unable to latch on to the breast. More often a baby starts out breastfeeding, but later begins struggling without success to latch on or simply refusing to nurse. Although his mother may think that he doesn't want to nurse, usually the baby wants to but can't. This problem can usually be identified and worked through.

The Baby Who Has Never Nursed. When trouble with latching on begins at the very first nursing, it can originate with either the mother or the baby. Flat, inverted, or dimpled nipples can make nursing difficult for a baby. Premature babies, and those who have been sick in the hospital, are sometimes sent home before breastfeeding has been established. Some babies have temporary problems with latching on to the nipple, coordinating normal sucking, or both. And bottle feeding can sometimes complicate the baby's nursing efforts.

If your baby hasn't latched on yet, rent a fully automatic electric breast pump so that you can collect your breast milk quickly and easily as well as keep up with your baby's milk needs. Use the pump every two to three hours during the day and evening, and whenever your baby awakens in the night. If you're using a single-collection kit, pump each breast twice for a total pumping time of about twenty minutes. A double-collection kit pumps both breasts simultaneously for a total pumping time of ten to twelve minutes.

If your baby has never latched on, you may be feeling very discouraged. If you have been working alone to get your baby nursing, here are some tips:

◆ Attempting to breastfeed at every feeding may be too frustrating, so limit your nursing sessions to once or twice a day.

◆ Try nursing your baby after a minute or so of pumping, when your nipple is more erect.

◆ Carefully review the latch-on technique outlined in the Appendix.

◆ Placing your thumb and index finger just behind your nipple and pressing—as if you are trying to make your fingers come together—will probably keep your nipple extended outward. Keep your fingers pressed together even when you pull your baby's mouth onto your nipple. Your fingers may be slightly inside the baby's lips; keep them there, continuing to hold your nipple firmly while your baby learns to grasp it.

◆ Dripping breast milk from a bottle over your nipple and into your baby's mouth (you might need a helper for this), or allowing her to suck on a finger (nail-side down), can also help to calm a crying baby and coax her to open her mouth in search of your nipple.

◆ If you are having problems maintaining your milk supply, see "Concerns about Your Milk Supply," page 36.

These suggestions are not guarantees to success, and certainly other problems not discussed here could be contributing to your struggle. A lactation professional can probably suggest techniques that may help you. Other sources of help or support may be found through a mother-to-mother support group such as La Leche League (see the Appendix).

Kathleen has seen many babies finally latch on after several weeks of persistent efforts. Occasionally, however, after a great deal of hard work it becomes clear that a baby is not going to breastfeed. If after six weeks of effort your baby still isn't latching on, it may be time to give up. Perhaps the combination of some underlying nipple or sucking problem with a few weeks of bottle feeding makes the baby unable or unwilling to nurse. You can, of course, continue to pump your milk and bottle-feed it to your baby, but this is twice the work of either breastfeeding or formula feeding. If you can't bear to continue this routine, weaning may be your only alternative.

The Baby Who Nursed Earlier but Now Refuses. The baby who has been nursing well but suddenly begins to refuse feedings is often a puzzle to his mother and even to health-care providers. If a baby has been getting bottles of formula daily (or almost daily) and his mother has not been expressing her milk during these skipped nursings, or if a breastfed baby has been getting daily supplemental bottles due to low milk supply or slow weight gain, he may begin to prefer the bottle (see "Concerns about Your Milk Supply," page 36). A baby who is not feeling well can lose interest in nursing, too. Have your baby's doctor examine him; if the doctor finds an illness—an ear infection, for example—be sure to express your milk frequently to maintain your supply. If no illness is diagnosed, there are still some steps you can take to remedy the situation.

Frequently Kathleen sees babies who, between the ages of about ten days and about three months, begin pulling off the breast, usually crying, and refusing to nurse. Mothers often say that these babies are happy to nurse at certain times, often in the middle of the night. These babies also tend to spit up frequently. Kathleen has observed that if the mother expresses her milk and puts it in a bottle, the baby will often happily take it. Why this is so remains unclear. But eliminating certain foods from the mother's diet often improves nursing within a few days.

If you suspect a food sensitivity, try eliminating all of the following from your diet, for two to three days: chocolate; fruits high in citric acid, such as oranges, lemons, limes, tangerines, grapefruit, kiwi fruit, strawberries, pineapples, and tomatoes; dairy products, such as milk, cheese, yogurt, sour cream, and ice cream; peanuts and peanut butter; and certain gas-producing vegetables (onions, cabbage, broccoli, Brussels sprouts, and cauliflower). Your baby may also be reacting to cow's milk or soy; eliminate any formula if your own milk supply is sufficient. For more information on food sensitivities, see "Dietary Intolerances," page 44.

Express your milk, using a fully automatic breast pump, as long as your baby refuses to nurse. Use the pump every two to three hours during the day and evening, and whenever your baby awakens in the night, for as long as he is not nursing.

Within three days your baby will probably be nursing better, and you can begin to reintroduce the suspected food categories to your diet, one every few days. For example, reintroduce a lot of dairy products for a day or two. If your baby responds well, try reintroducing citrus fruits on the next day, and so on. It can help to keep a food diary during this time. Your baby will probably show a negative reaction between two and eight hours after you have ingested an offending food.

If your baby has been refusing to nurse for some time, and you have been offering formula instead of expressing milk, things may be more complicated. Your milk supply may be too low to meet the baby's needs without supplementation. It is probably not too late to reverse this situation, however; see "Concerns about Your Milk Supply," below.

A "nursing strike"—a baby's sudden refusal to nurse for a few days—occurs most commonly between four and nine months of age. Although this behavior seems to occur without cause, it is usually associated with a respiratory or ear infection, or with teething, if a baby has bitten his mother and has been startled by her response. Some mothers decide to turn a nursing strike into a permanent weaning, but most can persuade their babies to resume nursing. For as long as your baby refuses to nurse, express milk frequently, preferably with a fully automatic breast pump. Try to give the milk by cup rather than by bottle, if possible, or you may only encourage the baby to continue refusing to nurse and to become dependent on the bottle.

Concerns about Your Milk Supply

The most frequent reason mothers give for weaning in the early months is that their milk is inadequate. Some mothers believe their milk is "weak" or in some other way lacking. Other mothers think they don't have enough milk. But breast-milk quality is relatively similar from mother to mother, even if a woman's diet is less than ideal, and only a small minority of mothers are incapable of establishing a normal supply of milk. Some mothers and babies struggle with a low milk supply during the first few weeks of breastfeeding because the breasts are not regularly stimulated and emptied. Birth-control pills containing estrogen, including the "low-dose" pill, can also diminish milk production (the "mini-pill," also known as the progestin-only pill, usually doesn't affect the milk supply). But the overwhelming number of mothers who think they have too little milk have babies who are taking plenty of milk and are gaining weight well. These mothers have based their conclusions on misinformation or a misinterpretation of their babies' behavior.

The best way to assess your milk supply is to have your baby weighed. A baby's weight gain indicates whether she is getting enough milk. Most home bathroom and baby scales are too imprecise, but you can either arrange to weigh your baby at her doctor's office (you shouldn't need an appointment to see the doctor, but do call ahead) or rent a lightweight electronic scale from a Medela pump-rental station. Weigh your baby just before a feeding, if possible, and without a diaper or other clothing.

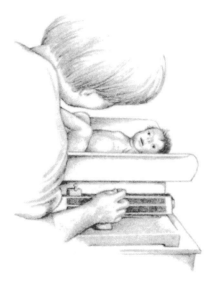

A newborn should have regained her birth weight by two weeks of age, and should gain close to an ounce a day thereafter for the first three to four months. If your baby was weighed any time after five days of age, use that weight to determine how much she has gained. For example, if at ten days of age your baby weighed 7 pounds, a week later she should weigh close to 7 pounds 7 ounces. If you haven't had your baby weighed for more than two weeks, you may be wise to weigh her twice, two or three days apart, for a more accurate indication of her current daily intake.

Your baby should gain about an ounce a day from two weeks until at least three months of age.

After three months of age a baby's weight gain may slow somewhat. A gain of at least one-half ounce a day usually indicates an adequate milk supply after the third month.

If you've been supplementing your milk with more than an ounce or two of formula per day, you cannot use your baby's weights alone to assess your milk supply. Assume that if a baby who has received supplements is gaining just an ounce a day, she probably needs the formula to continue gaining, until you increase your milk supply. But if your baby is gaining more than an ounce a day, she may not need the supplemental formula, or at least not as much of it (see "The Baby Who Is Not Gaining Enough or Who Is Receiving Supplements," page 39).

If your baby is receiving no supplements, and is gaining weight adequately but seems unsatisfied, consider one of several possible reasons. Perhaps you have certain expectations of how long and how often a baby should want to nurse. Most young babies want and need to nurse every one and a half to three hours around the clock. In the evening most babies are somewhat unsettled, and so may want to nurse much more often. Babies also tend to nurse with greater frequency at about two to three weeks of age and again at about six weeks. These appetite spurts may function to increase mothers' milk supplies for their babies' upcoming growth needs.

You may have been told that a baby empties the breast in ten minutes. But most young babies need to nurse for about fifteen to forty-five minutes at a time. Ending the feeding before the baby signals that she is finished—usually, by releasing the nipple herself—could leave her unsatisfied and fretful. It could also deprive her of the high-calorie milk that comes at the end of the feeding, so that she might want to nurse again sooner than she would otherwise.

Perhaps you have tried to express milk and have had trouble getting much, or maybe you're worried by how watery your milk looks. Most breast pumps, except for the fully automatic ones, are inefficient at stimulating and emptying the breast, and so shouldn't be used to evaluate milk production. And breast milk normally looks watery compared with cow's milk, especially at the start of a feeding. If you are expressing only the foremilk, perhaps because your pump doesn't bring out the hindmilk, you're not seeing the cream that increases near the end of a feeding.

Perhaps you are overwhelmed by the demands of your baby, and feel as if all you do is nurse. You might find it helpful to count the number of feedings in a twenty-four-hour period. Most young babies nurse between eight and twelve times a day. If your baby wants to nurse more than that, you might simply have a fussy infant who needs to nurse for comfort. (If she also spits up often, passes a lot of gas, or has more than eight stools per day or stools that are green in color, see "The Fussy Baby," page 44.)

If you have returned to work, you may be dealing with a low milk supply. When feedings are missed and milk is not expressed, or it is not expressed often enough to keep the breasts stimulated, a woman's milk supply will usually drop. Sometimes the problem is an inefficient pump, or a pump with an undersized nipple flange. When the nipple swells in response to suction, the milk flow is cut off if the tunnel of the flange is too narrow. It may be necessary to buy a flange with a wider tunnel. Best of all for correcting a low milk supply is a fully automatic breast pump (see page 29).

The Baby Who Is Not Gaining Enough or Who Is Receiving Supplements. If your baby is not gaining weight or is gaining less than he should, you may wonder if continuing to nurse your baby is a good idea. If you have been supplementing breast milk with formula every day, you may have doubts about which is best. Although any amount of breast milk is in a baby's best interest, the young baby who receives formula supplements will tend to wean sooner. Usually he takes more and more formula over time, and his mother's milk supply diminishes accordingly, until the baby begins to strongly prefer the bottle. This needn't happen. Even though a baby may need supplementation temporarily, a mother's low milk supply can often be reversed by increasing the amount of regular breast stimulation and emptying.

Certainly a baby who is not gaining enough weight should be examined by his doctor; some condition other than a low milk supply could be causing the low weight gain. Once your baby is cleared as healthy, you can work through this problem on your own, or you can get assistance from a lactation professional, who can evaluate your situation and recommend a course of action (see the Appendix for information on finding lactation professionals). Most health plans cover the cost of a consultation with a lactation professional, although some plans require a referral from a physician. Mother-to-mother support groups can also help in this situation.

The key to solving a problem of low weight gain is to understand how much milk your baby needs daily and how much milk you produce. With the guidelines that follow and, perhaps, the help of a lactation professional, you can estimate these amounts and then figure out how much supplementing is needed. If you have been supplementing with formula, you may be able to eliminate or cut back on its use by stimulating more breast milk production. Remember, however, that to abruptly stop giving a baby supplements without careful monitoring can be dangerous. When a baby has been receiving formula daily, especially if he has been getting more than 4 ounces a day, his mother may not be making enough milk for him to gain weight on without supplements.

Here is a simple way to estimate your baby's daily milk needs:

1. Weigh your baby, at least one hour after the last nursing (see page 37).

2. Convert his weight to ounces: Multiply the number of pounds by 16, and add any additional ounces.

3. Divide that number by 6. For example, a baby who weighs 8 pounds 3 ounces (131 ounces) would require 21.8, or approximately 22, ounces of milk per day (131 ounces divided by 6) in order to gain weight normally.

This formula must be based on your baby's current weight; you should recalculate it every week until your baby is gaining normally and any supplement has been eliminated.

Here is the way to estimate the amount of breast milk that you are producing:

◆ Use a fully automatic breast pump; anything less will not give you a true estimate. After one of your mid-morning nursings, use the pump to collect any milk left in each breast; pump both breasts for a total of about ten minutes.

◆ Put off nursing for the next two hours.

◆ Exactly two hours after the first pumping, use the electric pump again. At this time of day you are more likely to assess an average milk volume. Pump each breast, switching sides as your milk flow slows, and then pump each breast again; the entire pumping should take twenty to twenty-five minutes.

◆ Multiply the number of ounces collected at this second pumping by 12. The result represents approximately how much milk you are producing over a twenty-four-hour period. For example, if you collect 1½ ounces at the second pumping, you are producing about 18 ounces per day.

Now you can compare your baby's daily milk requirement with your actual milk production. For example, if you estimate that your baby needs 22 ounces a day and your milk production is 18 ounces per day, your baby needs 4 ounces of formula per day. You can offer the supplement after each nursing; just divide the total amount of supplement needed by the approximate number of daily feedings. In this example, if you feed the baby about nine times a day, you would give the baby one-half ounce of formula after each nursing. Or you could offer one ounce after only four or five of his daily nursings, perhaps in the afternoon and evening, when your milk production is slightly lower. The goal is to offer about the same amount of milk at each feeding so that your baby will want to nurse at regular intervals. After a week or so, re-estimate your baby's daily milk needs; because he will weigh more, his needs will have increased. Re-estimate your milk production at this time; it's likely that it, too, will have increased, so you can decrease or perhaps even eliminate the supplements.

Occasionally a mother determines that she has enough milk for her baby, and yet he does not gain well. Perhaps the baby is not taking all of the milk available at some or many of his feedings. This happens frequently with young babies who were born prematurely or who tend to drift off to sleep while nursing; with babies who have sucking difficulties; and sometimes with babies who are sensitive to something in the milk (see "The Fussy Baby"). In such a case you should consider pumping for a few minutes after most of your daytime nursings and offering your baby this milk by bottle after he nurses. Continue to monitor his weight closely until his nursing improves.

If you have been giving your baby supplements, and your estimates suggest that he needs less or more formula than you have been offering, make these adjustments slowly. Perhaps you started out giving your baby formula because you thought that he needed more milk, and now you estimate that you are making as much milk as he needs. In this case, cut the amount of supplement you are giving at feedings by half. In a few more days, decrease the amount again. You should be able to eliminate the supplement altogether in a week. If fussiness prompted you to supplement your baby's milk, read "The Fussy Baby," page 44. If you are worried about his milk intake, have your baby weighed; a gain of an ounce a day reflects an adequate milk intake.

If your baby is younger than three months, you may be able to increase your milk supply by increasing the number of feedings per day so that he nurses at least every two and a half hours (timed from the start of one nursing to the start of the next) during the day and evening and at least every five hours at night. Another effective way to stimulate your milk production is to switch your baby from one breast to another several times during a feeding. Nurse for as long as forty-five minutes, if he's willing. Remember to offer any supplement right after nursing.

Another technique for increasing a low milk supply is to use a fully automatic electric pump for five to ten minutes right after a feeding. Offer the milk to the baby, with any other necessary supplement, after he has nursed.

If your baby is older than three months and is not gaining weight, most likely his feedings have dropped below seven a day. By simply increasing the number of daily feedings, however brief they may be, you can build up your milk supply. Eliminate the pacifier, if your baby uses one, and offer your breast whenever your baby begins sucking his fingers. Some mothers increase their milk production by taking their babies to bed for a few days and nursing the time away. If your baby is older than four months, you could offer him solid foods (cereal mixed with breast milk; formula; fruits; and vegetables) after nursing, in addition to nursing more often.

Regardless of your baby's age, you may find fenugreek, a fragrant seed used in Indian cooking, to be very helpful in stimulating greater milk production. You can make tea from fenugreek seeds, but you may find it more convenient and more effective to take fenugreek capsules, which are sold in health-food stores. Women who take two to four capsules three times a day typically notice an increase in their milk production within one to three days. Fenugreek is harmless, although you will probably notice that your sweat and urine take on a distinct odor of maple. Rarely, a mother reports having diarrhea that quickly subsides when she stops taking fenugreek.

If your baby is not gaining weight adequately and you cannot use an electric pump to estimate your milk production, you can still improve your supply. The disadvantage of not knowing how much milk you are producing is that you can't be sure of how much formula to use as a supplement. Some babies take about as much formula as they need after they nurse, but others overconsume and are then less interested in nursing later—a situation that can lead to a further decline in the milk supply. You might consider weighing your baby frequently, every three or four days (see page 37). If he gains less than an ounce a day, he probably needs more milk or formula; if he gains more than an ounce a day, he could probably do with a little less.

If your milk production has been low for weeks, it may take quite a while to improve the situation. Some women find that they are simply unable to produce a full milk supply. This situation is usually evident from the first week of nursing. Many women who can't produce enough milk have had major breast surgery, such as a breast reduction or, sometimes, a breast augmentation, if the implant was inserted through the areola. Other women have insufficient glandular tissue; their breasts have simply never developed enough of the tissue in which milk is produced. In these women, typically, one breast is significantly smaller than the other and there is a large space between the breasts. The breasts don't change in fullness or in size during the early months of pregnancy or during the first three to five days postpartum, when milk normally comes in. Pumping with an electric breast pump rarely yields more than a few tablespoons of milk.

If you discover you can't produce enough milk, you may understandably want to wean quickly. You can still nurse if you wish, however, provided that you supplement your milk with formula. You might try a nursing supplementer—a small device that feeds formula through a thin, soft tube while the baby sucks at the breast (see the Appendix). Or you may enjoy nursing without a supplementer at times when your baby is not frantically hungry but just wants to suck.

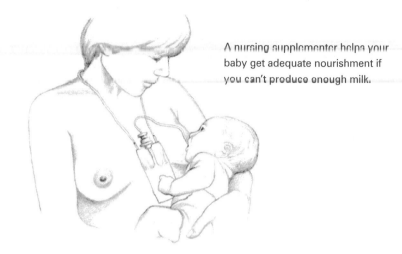

A nursing supplementer helps your baby get adequate nourishment if you can't produce enough milk.

The Fussy Baby

Many mothers who wean in the first four months seem to have made mistaken assumptions about their babies' behavior. Maybe you believe that your baby is unsatisfied, that she is getting too little milk, or that the milk does not agree with her. Maybe your baby wants to nurse all the time, or she frequently cries and fusses, or she has other symptoms, such as spitting up and vomiting, a stuffy nose, redness around the anus, excessive amounts of gas, or frequent, watery stools that may be green, bloody, or contain mucus. Some babies also pull off the breast crying or have rashes on the face and upper body. Often babies who have bouts of crying along with intestinal symptoms are labeled as colicky. Certainly your baby's doctor should rule out any other illness, but don't be surprised if he or she has no diagnosis other than colic. Although most colic symptoms usually resolve after a baby reaches three months of age, it isn't easy to have an unhappy baby and not know why. Even though you know that breast milk is best for babies in general, you may still wonder if your baby's symptoms and behavior mean that it's not best for her in particular. Fortunately, there are remedies less harsh than weaning for most discomforts that your baby may be experiencing.

Dietary Intolerances. Occasionally, foods or beverages in a mother's diet cause colic symptoms in her baby. If you have consulted the doctor about your baby's fussiness and perhaps even asked if something in your diet could be to blame, you've probably learned that the doctor has little to say about dietary intolerances in breastfed babies. Although some doctors are aware of one or two foods that can cause colic symptoms, most believe that colicky behavior has no connection to a mother's diet.

FRIDAY	
8:30 a.m. Orange juice Prenatal vitamin Oatmeal	
10:30 a.m. to 12:00 noon Toast with margarine	Fussy, spitting up
12:15 p.m. Ham and cheese sandwich 　(mustard and lettuce) Tortilla chips Milk	**2:00 to 5:00 p.m.** Crying
3:00 p.m. Pineapple-banana-orange juice	
6:45 p.m. Chicken-broccoli stir-fry Green salad with carrots 　(Italian dressing) Rice Milk	
8:15 p.m. Chocolate ice cream	**11:30 p.m. to 2:00 a.m.** Very fussy, vomited

Sample chart of a mother's diet and her baby's reactions

If your baby exhibits some or all of the symptoms described here every day or nearly every day, you may be able to pinpoint the cause by writing down everything you have eaten and drunk during the past three days, as shown in the sample chart for one day. Include any medications or vitamins that you take or give to the baby. Also make note of any particularly difficult periods for your baby during the past three days.

Be sure to consider other possible causes of fussiness. If you are producing a lot of milk, have your baby weighed to see how fast he is gaining. A baby who is gaining much more than an ounce a day might be having symptoms of hyperlactation syndrome (see "Overabundant Milk Supply," page 48). Be aware, too, that thrush can cause fussiness (see "Yeast Infections," page 49).

In most cases of dietary intolerance among breastfed babies, the culprits fall into one or more of several major food categories. The offending foods act either as intestinal irritants or as allergens. Often when a baby has specific periods of fussiness, the offending food can be identified by looking back one to two meal periods. If you completely eliminate all of the following food groups from your diet for three days, you could bring speedy relief to your fussy baby. Be sure to check the ingredients in any commercially processed food before you ingest it.

Chocolate. The major offender in chocolate is theobromide, a potent irritant to the digestive tract of many infants, even in small amounts. The chocolate ice cream listed in the chart was more than likely responsible for this baby's (and mother's) difficult night.

Acidic fruits. A frequently overlooked cause of digestive disturbances are citrus fruits and their juices. Oranges, lemons, limes, tangerines, and grapefruit can all bother a baby's intestines. Although tomatoes, pineapples, and strawberries are not citrus fruits, many babies respond similarly to them. Vitamin C supplements can produce colic symptoms, too. In the chart, the mother had orange juice at breakfast and another citrus beverage in the afternoon. Her baby may have been bothered by these.

Cow's milk. Some infants are allergic to cow's milk and cow's milk products, including cheese, yogurt, sour cream, butter, cottage cheese, and ice cream. If your baby is truly allergic to cow's milk, merely cutting back on your intake will probably not eliminate his symptoms. In this case, you must eliminate from your diet nearly all dairy products, including those in commercially processed foods such as creamed soups, salad dressings, and puddings; cow's milk might be identified as "casein" or "whey" on the label. (Don't worry if a milk product is a very minor ingredient—in a baked product such as bread, for example.) Many infant formulas are made from cow's milk, too. Weaning a baby who is allergic to cow's milk to a cow's-milk formula will almost certainly intensify his symptoms. Up to 50 percent of these babies will not tolerate soy formula, either. The mother's notes in the chart indicate that the baby may be reacting to dairy products.

Gas-producing vegetables. Certain vegetables—onions, broccoli, cauliflower, Brussels sprouts, cabbage, bell peppers, and cucumbers—can create temporary digestive problems for young babies. Prepared mustard can cause a similar reaction. Onions, an ingredient in so many dishes, can give a baby gas even when they are cooked, ingested in small amounts, or taken in the form of onion powder. The stir-fry dish listed in the chart contained some of these gas-producing foods.

One common cause of colic symptoms that is frequently overlooked is not a food, really, and it is routinely given directly to breastfed as well as bottle-fed babies. This substance is fluoride. Although fluoride is very helpful in preventing cavities, it may be best delayed until a baby is at least six months old. At least forego giving fluoride for the three days of your elimination diet.

During this time, too, continue to keep a dietary chart, noting your observations of your baby's behavior. If you notice any particularly difficult periods, look back one to two meal periods, or about two to eight hours, to try to identify any suspect foods. Maybe you ate something in the four categories without realizing it. Or perhaps a food outside of these categories is a problem. Foods that occasionally cause reactions include eggs (even the very small amounts in mayonnaise), peanuts and peanut butter, corn and corn syrup, wheat (in breads, crackers, cookies, cakes, and noodles), soy (the basis of some infant formulas and an ingredient in many processed foods), apples, and bananas. If you decide to eliminate any one of these food categories, continue to avoid the original four, too, since foods from more than one group could be causing your baby's symptoms.

If your baby is much better after the three days, with very few upset periods or other symptoms, try adding back milk products into your diet.

Have a lot of milk products early in the day, and then watch your baby for twenty-four hours. If the problems reappear, after a couple of days you might try experimenting with small amounts of various milk products, to see which of them, if any, your baby can tolerate. Although some babies cannot tolerate any milk products, some do fine when their mothers have hard cheese, and others can tolerate small amounts of any milk products as long as their mothers take them only once every few days. Every two or three days, add another food category to your diet, eating a lot at a time, preferably early in the day. If your baby's fussiness recurs, eliminate the offending food category from your diet again. Remember that more than one category of food can trouble a very sensitive baby.

Overabundant Milk Supply. If you are producing a lot of milk and your baby is gaining weight beyond the typical ounce a day, her colic symptoms could be caused by what some refer to as hyperlactation syndrome. This type of colic is characterized by gassiness, frequent stools, spitting up, and general discomfort and fussiness, but not by more obvious allergy symptoms like upper-body rashes and a stuffy nose (Woolridge and Fisher 1988). These babies show little improvement with a change in the mother's diet. They nurse frequently from both breasts, and their mothers have overabundant milk supplies.

The underlying cause of this type of colic is thought to be the baby's disproportionate intake of the low-fat foremilk, the milk that is available early in the feeding. When a baby consumes large amounts of foremilk and less of the fatty hindmilk, her stomach empties rapidly, dumping excess lactose into the bowel. This results in increased fermentation, gassiness, and discomfort.

To relieve this type of colic, get your baby to empty one breast completely at each feeding, so that she receives not only the foremilk but the hindmilk, too. Allow her to nurse from the first breast until, satisfied, she spontaneously pulls away; don't interrupt her by switching her over to the second breast. Some authorities feel that, until the colic subsides, the baby should be limited to one side for one and a half to two hours before nursing on the other side. Mothers report that they adjust easily to this method of nursing, and some say that their breasts feel more comfortable than when they were nursing on both breasts at each feeding.

Yeast Infections. Yeast infections, though common in infants, are frequently overlooked as the cause of excessive fussiness. A newborn can acquire a yeast infection while passing through the birth canal during delivery, or as a result of antibiotics given to either the baby or the mother (after a cesarean birth, for example, the mother may be given antibiotics in intravenous fluid). Antibiotics kill not only harmful bacteria, but also "friendly" bacteria that keep yeast from getting out of hand.

A baby with a yeast infection usually shows signs of thrush—white patches, sometimes on his tongue, but most typically on the inside of his lips and cheeks. Because the yeast is also frequently present in the intestinal tract, he will usually be very gassy. He may have a diaper rash, probably on and around the genitals, that may resemble a mild burn, or may be just a patch of red dots. The skin may peel, and ordinary diaper rash remedies don't help. The infection can spread to the mother's nipples, causing irritation, redness, and even painful cracks. To prevent recurrence, a yeast infection requires regular, thorough, and simultaneous treatment of both mother and baby according to the instructions under "Irritated and Burning Nipples," pages 30-32.

Plugged Ducts and Breast Infections (Mastitis)

Many nursing women experience plugged milk ducts, indicated by a sore area of the breast that doesn't soften with nursing. And up to 30 percent of all nursing mothers develop mastitis—that is, breast infection. Some women experience recurrent plugged ducts or mastitis, and many of them consider weaning for this reason.

Most common during the early weeks of nursing, plugged milk ducts can occur for a variety of reasons. Often a plugged duct follows a missed feeding or a long stretch at night without nursing. Bras that are too tight, especially those with underwires, obstruct milk flow, leading to plugged ducts; baby carriers with tight straps are another culprit. Although we don't know why, plugged ducts seem to occur more often during the winter months. Mothers with high milk production, including those nursing twins, seem to be more prone to plugged ducts. Some breastfeeding specialists say that drinking an insufficient amount of fluids, becoming slightly dehydrated due to a cold or other viral infection, or being overly fatigued can also increase a woman's susceptibility to plugged milk ducts.

A plugged duct can occur in one of the nipple openings, causing nipple pain. You may also notice an area of the breast that doesn't soften with nursing. If your nipple looks normal in color but has a white spot on its tip, particularly right after nursing, you may have a plugged nipple pore.

Like plugged milk ducts, mastitis occurs most often in the early weeks of nursing. Mastitis causes flu-like symptoms, including headache, fever, chills, aches, and sometimes nausea and vomiting. Normally only part of one breast is affected; it usually becomes hard, tender, and reddened. The redness may not be apparent until you look in the mirror. A breast infection may follow a cracked nipple or a plugged milk duct. All of the factors that lead to a plugged duct also can lead to mastitis. Prompt recognition of the oncoming signs—especially a headache, which often appears even before any breast tenderness is noticed—can often prevent more severe and prolonged symptoms.

To treat a plugged milk duct or mastitis, apply moist heat to the affected area just before nursing. Make sure your breast is frequently and completely emptied, by your baby or by a very effective breast pump. If the plugged duct is in the nipple, you can get rapid relief by gently opening the pore with a sterile needle (don't be alarmed if there is a little bleeding). If you have mastitis symptoms, consider calling your physician for an antibiotic, especially if moist heat and frequent nursing alone do not resolve your symptoms within twelve to twenty-four hours. Take the medication for at least ten days, even if the symptoms disappear after a day or two. (Be aware that a yeast infection can crop up during a course of antibiotics or any time within two weeks after the treatment is completed.) Acetaminophen (such as Tylenol) or ibuprofen (Advil, Motrin) will help reduce your fever and discomfort.

If you have a plugged milk duct or mastitis, this is not a good time to wean. A plugged milk duct can develop into mastitis, which in turn can worsen into an abscess, necessitating surgical drainage if the breast isn't frequently and completely emptied.

The multiple causes of recurrent plugged ducts and mastitis are poorly understood. Often plugged ducts and mastitis recur in women whose cracked nipples have healed without antibiotic treatment. Plugged ducts and mastitis also tend to recur when a baby doesn't completely drain the breast. If you have had episodes of either plugged ducts or mastitis, make sure that your baby drains at least one breast at every nursing. Don't interrupt the baby to switch him to the other side until he signals that he is finished; this is essential for mothers who produce a lot of milk. Also, avoid long stretches without nursing. If your baby sleeps in long stretches at night, you might express milk before you go to sleep, or in the morning after your baby nurses, to encourage more complete drainage.

If breast infections reappear in the same breast within two weeks, ask your physician about your antibiotic. Some antibiotics (such as Ampicillin) may not penetrate the breast tissue deeply enough to completely kill all of the bacteria. The drugs of choice for a breast infection include Dicloxicillin and, for mothers who are allergic to penicillin, Erythromycin and Keflex.

RETURNING TO WORK

Many women decide to wean their babies when they face returning to work. The typical workplace in the United States, unlike that in many other countries, does not make parenthood easy for employed mothers. When employed, most of us accept that any compromises to be made will be in the parenting side of our lives. Some mothers arrange to work on a flexible schedule, to work at home, or even to keep their babies at work. But most working mothers have no such privileges. Only a few states in this country protect women's right to breastfeed in the workplace; employers don't have to extend or change break times to accommodate breastfeeding mothers.

Yet more and more women today are combining employment and breastfeeding. Women who continue to nurse do so not only because of the health benefits that breastfeeding provides but also because they want to continue the intimate nursing relationship during the hours they are with their children. Practically speaking, babies who receive their mother's milk tend to be sick less often, so continuing to nurse may mean taking less time off work to care for a sick child. Nursing your baby during your time away from work is less of a hassle, and much less of an expense, than feeding formula.

Still, today's working-and-nursing mothers are pioneers. Returning to work is difficult enough with a young baby at home; making the arrangements necessary to continue breastfeeding complicates the matter. The following suggestions clarify the logistics involved in continuing to breastfeed, and present some options. You may decide that, through practical planning, you can overcome whatever obstacles you are anticipating.

Ideally, when a mother returns to work and her baby is still dependent primarily on her milk, she expresses her milk (or nurses, if she can arrange to do so) during breaks. This enables her to avoid engorgement, provide some or all of the milk that her baby requires, and, most important, maintain her milk supply. Accomplishing these goals requires four things: a place to express milk, the time to do so, an effective method for collecting milk, and a way to store the milk.

Perhaps you lack a private place to express your milk. If you don't have your own office, perhaps you can find another private area, such as a vacant office, lounge, storage area, or conference room. If the only available place is a lounge everyone uses at the same time, you might try to arrange your breaks for a different time. Your supervisor or a supportive coworker might help you come up with a creative solution. You may end up having to use the bathroom, but even this may be adequate so long as it is clean.

Maybe you feel you'll have no time to express milk, because your breaks and lunch period are irregular or brief. But it is not essential to express milk at the exact same time every day. Expressing milk two or three times during the work day, whenever you can manage it, will help maintain your supply.

If you've already tried pumping milk and found it difficult and time-consuming, consider trying a better pump. A good pump can make milk collection quick and easy. The manual and semiautomatic pumps sold in stores and catalogs, although fine for occasional pumping, are inefficient for everyday use at work. Manual pumps require repetitive pulling of a plunger or a cylinder (and use of both hands); semiautomatic pumps, whether battery-operated or plug-in, require repetitive movement of a finger on a button, or on a small opening, in order to create and release the suction.

To get the most milk in the least amount of time, to maintain full milk production, and to do so easily and comfortably, you'll want to rent or purchase a fully automatic breast pump (see page 29). With one of these, you can even eat, drink, or get some work done while you pump. If you also buy a double-collection kit, you'll need only ten to twelve minutes to pump—even if you have had trouble getting your milk to let down with another pump. Fully automatic pumps are available through thousands of rental stations and retail outlets across the country (see the Appendix). Renting one costs just $30 to $50 a month, far less than formula. Buying one, such as the Pump In Style or Purely Yours, costs about the same as two to three months' supply of formula.

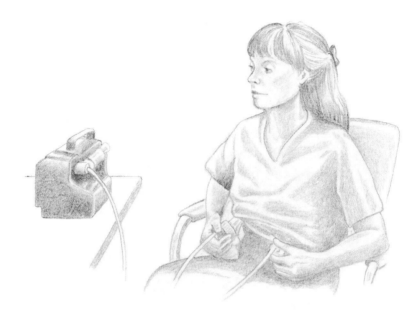

If you are frequently on the road, or have no electrical outlet where you pump, these pumps can run off a separate battery pack or plug into a car's cigarette lighter with an adapter (see the Appendix).

Although most women who nurse while employed away from home use some type of pump for collecting milk, some women quite effectively express milk by hand and find this to be a more convenient and natural method. To rely on manual expression, you'll need to practice before you return to work. Position your thumb and index finger about one and a half to two inches behind the nipple, where the milk sinuses are located. Push your fingers back toward your chest and press them together with a rolling motion, lifting the nipple outward; avoid sliding your fingers from their original position. Once you have the motion down, rotate your fingers around the nipple to empty other milk sinuses. With several practice sessions, most mothers can master manual expression. At work you may even be able to express both sides at the same time.

Storing your milk is easier than you might think. Expressed milk can be stored in any clean container. A lot of mothers use the disposable plastic liners from various bottle-feeding systems. Twist, bend, and secure the top of the bag with a rubber band or twist tie; then refrigerate it or place it in a small cooler or insulated container along with a refreezable ice pack. Breast milk can be refrigerated for as long as five days or kept frozen for three months.

You may worry about engorgement and leaking milk at work, especially if you must go long periods without expressing milk. If you can't express milk more often, wear nursing pads to prevent wet clothing (keep extra pads at work). The plastic breast shells available through some maternity shops and catalogs can be worn in place of pads to hold leaking milk, but keep in mind that they may encourage further leaking. A new product called LilyPadz, thin pads made of silicone, keeps the breasts from leaking at all. See the Appendix for information on finding these products. Or avoid embarrassment simply by wearing loose, light-colored tops and keeping an extra shirt, jacket, or sweater at work. When your milk starts to let down, crossing your arms against your chest for a few seconds will probably stop the leaking until you are able to express milk or nurse your baby. Leaking milk typically lessens and, eventually, stops as the weeks go by.

Maintaining an adequate milk supply is important for women who choose to return to work without weaning. A good milk supply depends on frequent stimulation and emptying of the breasts—at least seven to eight times in twenty-four hours. When the breasts are stimulated less frequently than this—whether by nursing or by expressing milk—the milk supply is liable to dwindle until it can no longer meet the baby's needs. This means you should nurse your baby as often as possible when you are together, so you can keep to a minimum the time you spend expressing. If your baby sleeps through the night, you might want to pump before you go to bed or very early in the morning. You might encourage night feedings by sleeping with your baby; neither of you will have to waken fully to nurse.

You might also try taking fenugreek, which some mothers have found is very helpful in stimulating increased milk production (see page 42). Fenugreek is usually used for a brief period of time to boost a low milk supply, but some mothers have continued to use it for much longer periods without problems. You may need to rely on a little formula as well when you are apart from your baby.

When you are anticipating a return to work or school, it is best to offer the baby a bottle of breast milk beginning at about three to four weeks of age. Offer her an ounce or two once or twice a week to keep her accustomed to the bottle. Offering a bottle much earlier or more often than this is unnecessary, and could interfere with your milk supply and your baby's interest in nursing. If you're going to be giving your baby formula, you may have to mix it in increasing proportions with breast milk until she no longer objects to the taste.

> Introduce a bottle at about three to four weeks of age, and offer one once or twice a week thereafter until you go back to work.

A baby who has never had a bottle and is older than one month, or who has gone weeks without a bottle, may strongly object to the whole idea. For helpful tips, see "Getting Your Baby to Take a Bottle," page 73.

If you definitely don't want to express milk while at work or you are unable to do so, you can still continue to nurse your baby in the morning and evening, at night, and during your days off, and you can provide formula for the times you are away from her. Part-time nursing works best if the baby is older than six months and is well established on other foods, or if she misses only a few nursings a week. Assuming that she can tolerate formula, if your baby is younger than six months or you are working full time (or close to it), your decision not to express milk may still present two difficulties: engorgement at work and a dwindling milk supply.

Engorgement can be uncomfortable and may lead to leaking milk, but after a short period of inadequate breast stimulation milk production usually slows and this problem fades. The bigger problem is the slowing of milk production, which can lead to a baby's unwillingness to continue nursing some or most of the time when she and her mother are together. Ultimately, the baby may wean herself. If she does, of course, she still has benefited from getting her mother's milk for a while longer than she would have if she had been weaned before her mother's return to work.

BUSINESS TRIPS, VACATIONS, AND HOSPITALIZATION

If you are anticipating a separation from your baby of a few days or longer, you may look at weaning as a necessity. But there may be an alternative.

If you are planning an upcoming trip, you can rent an electric breast pump (see the Appendix), and pump to maintain your milk supply while you and your baby are separated. Your baby can receive formula while you are gone, or you can rent the pump a couple of weeks before your trip and collect some or all of the milk that he will need by expressing extra milk right after nursings.

Although you may not be able to pump milk while away quite as often as you would normally be nursing, you should pump as often as possible throughout the day and evening. You'll probably toss out most of the milk, but you might consider refrigerating the milk from the last couple of days of your trip and carrying it home in a small cooler along with frozen ice packs (if you are staying in a hotel, the staff will probably be happy to freeze the ice packs for you). When you return home, place the milk in your freezer for later use. If you find that your milk supply has lessened upon your return, a few days of stepped-up nursing will increase your production.

Hospitalization of a nursing mother rarely necessitates weaning, although some doctors do advise it. Some hospitals have electric breast pumps available for nursing mothers; if yours doesn't, you can rent a pump and take it with you, or have one brought in. You may be able to arrange for your baby to be brought in for nursing visits, or even to stay with you (so long as you, a family member, or a friend can care for him).

If you are expressing your milk in the hospital, try to do so frequently to maintain your milk supply. Ask the nursing staff to refrigerate your milk so that it can be taken home for your baby.

If questions arise about the safety of medications you take in the hospital, see "Medications," page 63. If you must take a drug that is considered unsafe for a nursing baby, continue to pump your milk in order to maintain your supply, but discard the milk until the medication is no longer necessary.

If your milk supply drops while you are in the hospital, more frequent pumping or stepped-up nursing once you arrive home should reverse the situation in a few days. Review "Concerns about Your Milk Supply," page 36.

JEALOUS MATE

Few couples are totally prepared for the changes in a relationship that accompany the birth of a child. The baby, her care, and her feeding absorb a tremendous amount of time, especially during the early weeks. A mother naturally becomes quite preoccupied with her baby, and she does not always have energy left over for other things. Most new mothers need a great deal of support, and many need their mates to provide this for them. A mother may look to her mate to take over household chores, to help care for the baby, and, perhaps most important, to express interest and concern about herself and the baby. When a woman's primary focus shifts from her mate to her baby, however, her mate may feel displaced and neglected. Lack of time and fatigue can cause feelings of isolation on both sides. If your private time with your mate seems to have disappeared, you may wonder whether your relationship can survive your new baby's demands. And you may wonder if weaning could make things better.

Weaning to a bottle will not necessarily decrease the amount of time you spend caring for your baby. Although both you and your mate may at times feel tired, overwhelmed, and upset, understand that most new parents experience these emotions during the early weeks or months, regardless of the feeding method they have chosen. Your baby's demands will lessen considerably as she gets older and you become more confident in caring for her. In the meantime, if you think that you and your mate could benefit from more time together, then plan for some. Consider an occasional evening out without the baby; if you prefer not to leave her behind, select a restaurant that caters to families or plan a daytime outing. A family walk or drive can provide for some uninterrupted communication.

Not only may you and your mate lack time to talk together without interruption, but your sex life may be suffering as well. Fatigue and lack of time may dampen desire for both of you. Breastfeeding may provide all the physical attention you yourself need, leaving you feeling "touched out" at the end of the day. Maybe the physical changes in your body have also affected your feelings about sex. Intercourse may be uncomfortable because of tenderness from childbirth and hormonal changes that inhibit vaginal lubrication. Fears of another pregnancy can color your feelings about sex (see "Birth Control," page 63). And you may feel disappointed or even resentful that you still don't have your old body back. Perhaps you don't feel sexy; your breasts may seem more functional than erotic. Your mate may also have difficulty sorting out his feelings about your body now that you have given birth and are breastfeeding.

Many women worry about the changes in their feelings about sex, but generally these feelings are temporary. Breastfeeding isn't entirely to blame for these, either; bottle-feeding mothers also have sex less frequently after giving birth. Talking your feelings through can help both you and your mate feel reassured about this period in your relationship. And although you may not have the time and energy for intercourse, you can still enjoy cuddling and kissing. Being verbally affectionate can also help to rekindle warm feelings between you. When you want to have sex, don't be shy about planning for it.

Maybe you worry that your mate feels excluded from the mother-child relationship. How will he "bond" with the baby, you may wonder, if he can't feed her? Certainly a father needs opportunities to develop a relationship with his child, but this doesn't necessitate his feeding her. Actually, although some fathers like giving a bottle now and then, most appreciate not having to share the responsibility of full-time bottle feeding, especially in the middle of the night. It may help you both to understand that most babies prefer their mothers at first. This preference normally shifts back and forth between parents as the child grows.

Your mate can become involved with your baby by bringing her to you to nurse, and by burping, changing, and bathing her. During feedings, your mate can bring you something to drink, and even feed you while you nurse. He can care for the baby himself while you tend to your own needs; this will not only help him develop a relationship with the child, but will also help him understand some of the demands on you.

If you want your baby to have an occasional bottle because you're planning to go back to work or school, your mate can certainly feed her. Have your mate give the baby expressed breast milk from a bottle once or twice a week; this will keep her from refusing the artificial nipple later. (Remember, however, that it is best not to start offering a bottle before three to four weeks of age, or to delay it until much after one month of age.)

The demands of housework can add to the strain on a couple's relationship. Trying to keep a home perfectly clean and organized can leave you frustrated and exhausted. Some new mothers try each day to accomplish one household task—washing a load of laundry or a pile of dishes—so they can feel they've done something besides taking care of the baby. This is a reasonable goal, but a perfectly tidy home is not. If your mate complains about the mess, you may feel really inadequate—or really angry. Again, talking over your feelings should help. Try to agree on some reasonable standards of tidiness, and let your mate take on a bigger share of the chores.

CRITICAL FAMILY AND FRIENDS

Family members and friends can have a tremendous effect on your success at nursing and caring for your baby. Whereas some of your friends and relatives may be very supportive, others may interfere or offer subtle or even blatant criticism. Some comments may reflect a misunderstanding of how breastfeeding works; many new mothers endure hints that their diets are inadequate for milk production, and reports that other family members "didn't have enough milk," had "bad milk," or had milk that was "unsatisfying" for their babies. Other comments may reflect values from the past, when formula feeding was seen by middle-class women as scientific and modern ("I don't know why you bother with nursing; I bottle-fed you, and you turned out just fine").

However well-intentioned, a friend or relative who raised her children on formula may say inappropriate things because she knows nothing helpful to say. She may simply wish to help you out of a seemingly frustrating situation.

You may wonder if these people are right that breastfeeding is foolish or just too difficult. Or you may feel terribly alone; if you wean, you may think, at least you'll be normal. If you want to keep breastfeeding, though, it's important to get support especially in the early weeks of breastfeeding, when you are most vulnerable. Voice your needs to whoever can best meet them—your mate, a friend or relative who has breastfed, or a breastfeeding counselor. Once you have more confidence and experience, you will be able to handle the comments, opinions, and criticisms so frequently offered to nursing mothers.

FEELING TIRED, UNPRODUCTIVE, AND ISOLATED

Fatigue is one of the most common complaints of new mothers. To give birth and then immediately be put on call twenty-four hours a day can leave you physically and emotionally exhausted. Your fatigue is probably even worse if you are struggling with a fussy baby, breastfeeding complications, or other family demands. Tiredness can affect your emotions, your physical recovery, and your ability to reason; it can also affect your relationships with your mate and other children, leading to irritability and arguments.

The fatigue that follows childbirth seems to be universal among mothers regardless of their feeding method. Breastfeeding, however, means that you alone are responsible for every feeding. A few mothers find that having someone else give an occasional bottle of expressed breast milk or formula allows them a little extra sleep, but many women find that this is not an easy option: They don't want to interrupt their mates' sleep; their full breasts don't respond well to a skipped feeding; or they are afraid an occasional bottle would lower the milk supply.

To reverse fatigue, you need to slow down and get extra rest, especially during the early weeks. Napping with your baby during the day, and taking him to bed with you at night, may keep you from getting exhausted. You must also realize that you will not have the time or energy for all of those other things that you used to do so easily.

Feeling unproductive can be frustrating, especially if during pregnancy you fantasized about all the things you would accomplish while you were at home with your baby. You can get a few things done, though, without wearing yourself out. If you carry your baby in a cloth sling or pack when he is awake, you can keep him happy while you clean up the house or take a stroll. Later, when he's ready to nurse, you can feel good about relaxing with him. You'll also have one arm free to hold the phone or turn the pages of a book—something bottle-feeding mothers miss.

Still, for a while you're bound to spend most of your time caring for your child. Mothers least bothered by this situation are perhaps most convinced of the worth of full-time parenting. For them a baby's healthy growth and development reflect the important hours spent holding and nursing him. Finding friends who think this way will help, as will remembering that your situation is temporary: As your baby grows and matures, his care, nursing included, will get a lot less demanding.

As you adjust to the magnitude of your new job as a mother, you may find yourself feeling housebound and lonely. Caring for a baby can make you feel tied to the home. Getting out without the baby for more than two or three hours means not only finding someone else to care for him, but also expressing milk or providing formula, and hoping the baby will take the bottle. And when you do leave the baby behind, you may find yourself missing him or worrying about him. This can happen even after weaning.

Getting out of the house with the baby can be difficult, too. A stroller can help; a sling or front-pack may be even better, especially if you use public transportation. The weather, of course, can deter you for days or weeks. Still, taking a walk, visiting with friends, or going shopping can be a welcome change from your isolation at home. And taking a nursing baby along means not having to lug around bottles and figure out how to keep the formula cold and warm it up.

Nursing when you're out with the baby may make you anxious, especially during the early weeks when you and the baby are less experienced with latch-on. Women deal with nursing in public in a variety of ways. Some mothers respond to the baby without hesitation; others retreat to a private spot; and some get the baby started in private and then return once he is settled at the breast. Some mothers simply won't nurse in front of others; they bring along a bottle of expressed breast milk or formula instead.

If you're uncomfortable nursing around other people, choose tops that you can lift up from the bottom to expose less of you. Practice discreet latch-on techniques in front of a mirror or your mate or friend. In a restaurant, select a seat facing away from other diners. Locate comfortable bathrooms (with chairs), private lounges, dressing rooms, or other out-of-the-way places where you can sit and nurse. With time and experience, most women become more comfortable with public nursing.

If none of your old friends have children, overcoming loneliness may mean establishing new social circles. Coworkers and other acquaintances with whom you have had little in common may turn into fast friends when you discover how much you share as mothers. You might find friends, too, among the people you met in your childbirth class. Joining a new moms' or La Leche League group can provide an instant social support network. You might also look for a baby-sitting co-op in your area, or organize one yourself. Once you're comfortable taking your baby out in the world, you may discover that your social life is richer than ever.

WET CLOTHES AND UGLY BRAS

Leaking milk is common during the early weeks of nursing. Some women are constantly wet during these weeks, and some continue to leak for long afterward. When your milk lets down—because it's time to feed the baby, or you're already nursing, or your breast is stimulated in some other way—milk is released into the sinuses behind the nipple. Until the muscular ring behind the nipple is fully functional, milk can leak, drip, or spray.

Leaking breasts can be annoying and sometimes embarrassing. You may want to wear nursing pads until the leaking becomes more predictable or stops entirely. The cost of disposable pads adds up, of course; washable cotton pads, either purchased or homemade, may be more economical. They may also be more comfortable, and if they're contoured they'll look more natural under your bra than disposable pads would. At night, when you may leak more because your baby nurses less, you can protect your mattress with a waterproof mattress pad, and your bedding with a bath towel.

It is often possible to control leaking, to some extent, during the day. When the milk lets down, you may be able to prevent leaking by gently pressing against your nipples with your wrist or forearm for a few seconds (you can do this discreetly around other people by crossing your arms). Or try LilyPadz, thin silicone pads worn against the breasts to prevent leaking. If you have a lot of milk and your baby is gaining weight well, you might consider reducing leaking by nursing on just one breast per feeding. Whether you try this or not, be assured that the problem will diminish considerably with time.

Although nursing bras are not a necessity, most mothers find them convenient, particularly during the early weeks. They provide support, easy access for nursing, and a way to secure a nursing pad. You may view nursing bras with the same disdain you probably developed for maternity clothes; thankfully, these bras have become more attractive in recent years.

Still, you may long for something else. A stretch bra that you can pull up or down for nursing, or a regular bra that opens in front, will probably work well. Keep in mind that underwire bras have been associated with plugged milk ducts and breast infections. If you don't need nursing pads and you are more comfortable without a bra, there is no reason to wear one; going without a bra doesn't cause sagging breasts.

MEDICATIONS

You may think you have to wean your baby because you need to take a medication. Although most medications pass into breast milk, they do so in very small amounts, and most are safe for the nursing infant. It's important to get up-to-date information on any medication you must take, even an over-the-counter variety. Unfortunately, many health-care professionals lack knowledge about the effects of drugs in breast milk. An emergency-room doctor, internist, or other physician might tell you that a medication necessitates weaning—or that it is perfectly safe for your baby—without really knowing that this is true. *The Physician's Desk Reference* and drug- package inserts are poor sources of information on the effects of drugs in breast milk. Your baby's doctor may be able to find out for sure if a drug is safe. If not, try a lactation professional or a drug-information service (see the Appendix).

If you must temporarily take a medication that poses a risk to your baby, you can express your milk and discard it until you're off the drug. A fully automatic breast pump will make this work quicker, easier, and more comfortable than most other pumps could, and will better maintain your milk supply (see the Appendix to locate a rental pump). Use the pump every two to three hours during the day and evening, and whenever your baby awakens at night.

If you must take indefinitely a medication considered unsafe for nursing babies, be sure to learn what, if any, alternative drugs or treatments are available, and confirm this information with more than one source. Don't let your baby be needlessly weaned because of mistaken assumptions or misinformation.

BIRTH CONTROL

Many women consider weaning because they want the reliable and convenient birth control that "the pill" provides. Although hormonal birth control apparently does no direct harm to a nursing baby, pills containing estrogen, even in low doses, often reduce a mother's milk supply and result in underfeeding. Fortunately, not all birth-control pills interfere with milk production. The progestin-only pill, known as the "mini-pill," has no effect on milk supply, nor do progestin-only injections (which give three months' protection against pregnancy) or Norplant subdermal implants. Other birth-control methods, including foam, sponges, condoms, IUDs, diaphragms, cervical caps, and surgical sterilization, are also considered safe for the nursing baby.

The reliability of any of these birth-control methods is increased by the fact that you are breastfeeding. For now, in fact, breastfeeding may be the only birth-control method you need. That breastfeeding affects fertility is a truth that has been largely ignored in an era in which partial breastfeeding and early weaning have been the norm. But breastfeeding provides protection against more unwanted pregnancies worldwide than all other birth-control methods combined. Frequent nursing, especially during the baby's first several months, tends to suppress ovulation. In fact, exclusive breastfeeding in a mother who has not yet had a period provides more than 98 percent protection against pregnancy during the first six months postpartum (Kennedy et al. 1989).

When your baby begins to take food and drink other than your milk, when your periods resume, or when your baby reaches six months of age, your chances of getting pregnant increase, and you should not rely on breastfeeding alone for contraception.

DOCTOR'S ADVICE

Perhaps a doctor has suggested that you wean your baby. Since you're probably seeing your baby's doctor regularly during your child's early months, you may naturally turn to the doctor for advice on baby care, growth, infant behavior, and breastfeeding. Although most doctors believe in the benefits of breastfeeding, few are experts on this topic. More and more pediatricians and family practitioners are female, and those who have breastfed can share advice from their own experience. But few doctors have received much instruction about breastfeeding, and some doctors simply don't have the time to provide in-depth information and support for new parents.

Many nursing mothers voice disappointment with their doctors' lack of support, and, frankly, many doctors give bad advice on breastfeeding.

Maybe your doctor has recommended that you limit feedings, either in duration or frequency. Such advice, while intended to help you avoid soreness or get more rest, is contrary to successful nursing. The physician may even have advised you to stop nursing, assuming, perhaps, that if you asked whether your milk could be to blame for your baby's fussiness, you wanted permission to wean. Or maybe the doctor simply does not know how to help except by recommending formula supplements or complete weaning.

Even when a problem is more concrete than fussiness, a doctor may neglect to investigate the causes. Recently a young mother called Kathleen's clinic for assistance in weaning her two-month-old, who had become fussy and had been gaining weight poorly since his one-month checkup. The pediatrician, whom the mother believed to be supportive of breastfeeding, had suggested formula without inquiring about possible causes of the baby's poor weight gain. In response to Kathleen's questions, the mother reported that her obstetrician had started her on a low-dose estrogen birth-control pill at her six-week postpartum visit. Her baby's poor weight gain and unhappiness, then, were probably due to the estrogen, which inhibits milk production.

None of this means that you should necessarily look for another doctor if yours suggests formula, or that you shouldn't consider your doctor's opinions. It is important that you have a good physician and accurate information about breastfeeding. But you may not find both in the same person. If you feel confident in your doctor's medical skills, you needn't change doctors. But before deciding to wean because of a doctor's advice, find another source of guidance. You can get the information and support you need from a La Leche League leader or other breastfeeding counselor, an experienced nurse or childbirth educator, or a lactation professional (see the Appendix).

How to Wean Your Young Baby

If you are clear in your decision to stop nursing, you have many things to consider: how quickly to proceed; what type of formula to use; how to get your baby to accept a bottle; how to prepare formula; how much formula to give; and how to establish a good feeding relationship.

WEANING GRADUALLY OR ABRUPTLY

Slow weaning is generally easier on both mother and baby, and this is especially so in the early months. Most mothers of young babies have established large milk supplies that cannot be instantly shut down. Weaning over a period of two weeks or more allows a mother to avoid engorgement as she slowly reduces her milk production, and to observe her baby's tolerance for formula before the milk is gone. In addition, the level of immunological substances in breast milk increases with gradual weaning, offering the baby extra protection against infection as breastfeeding slowly comes to an end. Sometimes mothers begin gradual weaning only to discover that nursing less often is pleasurable, and so they continue on with partial breastfeeding.

If you must wean quickly, you can still evaluate your baby's response to formula before you've lost your milk. Feed formula exclusively for several days or more, and express your milk during this time (a fully automatic electric breast pump can make expressing your milk easier and faster). You can freeze the milk for the baby to have after the test period is over.

A baby who can't tolerate her formula will show any or all of these symptoms: bouts of crying, a lot of gas, increased spitting up or vomiting, body rashes, redness around the rectum, and frequent watery stools that may be green, bloody, or contain mucus (soy formulas typically produce pale-green, semi-formed stools). Wheezing and a stuffy or runny nose can also be allergic responses to formula.

If your baby does not seem to tolerate cow's-milk formula, check with your doctor about switching to a soy formula. Be aware, though, that about a third to half of all babies who are allergic to cow's-milk formulas are also allergic to soy formulas. If your baby doesn't tolerate soy, your

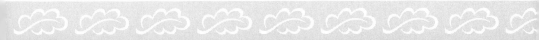

next option may be one of the hypoallergenic "predigested" formulas, which are very expensive. More than a few mothers who have weaned in the early months have regretted it when they've realized that their babies can't tolerate ordinary formulas. Some mothers have even tried relactating, which can be difficult. This is why you should either wean slowly or keep up your milk supply by pumping until you are sure that your baby can tolerate formula.

Weaning all at once or over a period of just a few days can threaten a mother's health as well as her baby's. Mothers who wean abruptly often suffer from breast pain caused by engorgement, which can last for several days until the breasts stop producing milk. Abrupt weaning can also lead to "milk fever"—mild fever, headache, general aching, and fatigue, typically lasting three to four days, and thought to be caused by the reabsorption of milk into the body. Milk fever is not the same as a breast infection, or mastitis, which also occasionally occurs during weaning. Mastitis is distinguished by a reddened area of the breast together with flu-like symptoms. Whereas milk fever resolves without treatment, mastitis following weaning usually requires antibiotic therapy.

If you must wean quickly, there are various things you can do to minimize or relieve engorgement. First, you can nurse or express just enough milk to keep you comfortable (unless you are taking an unsafe medication, you should give any milk you collect to your baby). Letting your breasts remain full will allow substances in the milk, called suppressor peptides, to inhibit further milk production. A supportive bra, a mild pain reliever, and ice packs can relieve the discomfort of engorgement. Some lactation professionals recommend chilled cabbage leaves, a very old remedy. Wearing the leaves inside your bra—and changing them periodically with fresh-chilled ones from the refrigerator—may decrease your swelling and discomfort. You might also hasten the decline of milk production with another engorgement remedy, sage tea: Steep 1½ teaspoons dry sage leaves in a pint of freshly boiled water for ten minutes. Drink as many as three cups a day, but continue this regimen for no longer than a week. Finally, you might try using vitamin B_6 (pyridoxine) to suppress lactation. Taking two 100-milligram tablets three times a day for the first day, and one tablet daily thereafter, can speed the process of drying up, although possible side effects include nausea, vomiting, diarrhea, and dark yellow-colored urine.

After rapid weaning, your breasts may feel full and lumpy for five to ten days. Unless you also have mastitis symptoms, this should be no cause for concern. The lumps will go away.

You may wonder about using "dry-up" medications to end milk production. Until recently, these drugs were frequently prescribed in maternity wards for mothers who did not intend to breastfeed. Although some doctors still prescribe the drugs, they have potentially serious side effects. Women who have taken Parlodel, the most common dry-up drug, have suffered seizures and strokes, and some of them have died (although the maker of Parlodel is no longer marketing it as a lactation suppressant, some doctors may still prescribe it for this purpose). These drugs are also quite expensive, and they take a few days to have an effect. In the meantime, the engorgement that naturally occurs probably makes milk production decline, anyway. And, after a ten-day course of the medication, milk production sometimes actually resumes.

When a mother must bring milk production to an immediate end, as is sometimes necessitated by a serious medical condition, a doctor might prescribe Dostinex (cabergoline). A one-time dose of 1 milligram Dostinex brings about rapid and complete cessation of milk production. Although Dostinex has not been approved by the U.S. Food and Drug Administration to suppress lactation, the drug is used for this purpose in Europe, and initial clinical trials in the United States indicate that this medication causes fewer side effects, such as headache, dizziness, and nausea, than other drugs used to halt milk production. Dostinex may cause a slight lowering of blood pressure.

More gradual weaning has no hard and fast rules. In the weaning process are two main steps: substituting something else for each nursing, and watching for any physical or emotional reactions in your baby or yourself. You can begin weaning by replacing a day or evening nursing with a formula feeding. If you observe no reactions to the formula—such as rash, increased spitting up or vomiting, bowel problems, crying bouts, wheezing, or nasal congestion—and if you don't feel engorged, after a few days or weeks you can replace a second nursing. The last feedings you'll replace will probably be the early morning and sleep-time nursings. Ideally, the pace of weaning occurs slowly enough to avoid causing an unhappy, clingy baby or full, uncomfortable breasts. (If at any time during the process you notice that your baby is not tolerating the formula,

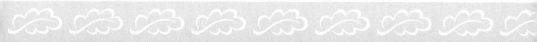

or if you simply miss nursing and change your mind about weaning, several days of stepped-up nursing will probably rebuild your milk supply. See "Concerns about Your Milk Supply," page 36.)

Even if you wean gradually, you may experience engorgement after you eliminate the last nursing or two. Again, a supportive bra, a mild pain reliever, ice packs, cabbage leaves, and sage tea may all help (see page 67). You can also relieve engorgement with an occasional brief nursing or by expressing small amounts of milk as needed. You may experience a few days of "milk fever" (see page 67). Again, watch for signs of a breast infection.

Regardless of whether you wean quickly or slowly, your fertility will probably return when you stop nursing, if not before. Any decrease in milk production during the weaning process can stimulate ovulation. For most women, fertility returns within a month or two after complete weaning.

SELECTING A FORMULA

Unless you have already offered your baby a certain formula that he seems to tolerate, you may be unsure of which one to try. There is no one "best" formula. Formulas come in three basic varieties—cow's milk, soy, and "predigested" or hypoallergenic. Your baby's doctor will probably recommend a cow's-milk formula unless there is reason to suspect that your baby has an allergy to cow's milk. If another family member has a milk allergy, or if your baby reacted to dairy products in your diet during breastfeeding, try one of the soy formulas instead. "Predigested" formulas, which are quite expensive, are intended for those infants who don't tolerate either cow's milk or soy.

A few companies produce most of the formulas you'll see in the market. Which brand you choose makes little difference. If your baby's doctor or the office nurse is loyal to a certain company, this probably has little to do with the quality of that company's formula.

Formula made from cow's milk is available in either low-iron or iron-fortified forms. Soy formulas are all iron-fortified. Iron-fortified formulas are believed to prevent iron deficiency, the most common cause of anemia in childhood. Iron deficiency has also been associated with subtle behavioral differences that cannot be corrected with iron supplements later on.

The American Academy of Pediatrics recommends that iron-fortified formula be used for all formula-fed babies. Still, low-iron formula remains available because some doctors believe that iron-fortified formulas are more likely to cause gastrointestinal problems, such as colic, constipation, diarrhea, spitting up, and vomiting. This belief is contradicted by numerous studies.

For various reasons, including cost, some mothers express interest in feeding goat's milk, plain cow's milk, or homemade formulas. None of these are as good as commercially manufactured formulas, and some homemade formulas can be dangerous. Regular pasteurized cow's milk, whether it is whole, low-fat, or skim, should not be introduced before a baby reaches one year of age. Feeding a baby cow's milk, a poor source of iron, can lead to iron-deficiency anemia. The excessive protein in cow's milk can put too great a load on a baby's kidneys. Because plain milk, even if pasteurized, has not been heated to the high temperatures used in manufacturing formulas, it is harder to digest and can cause intestinal blood loss. Cow's milk is also deficient in vitamins C and E and copper. Goat's milk is less allergenic than cow's milk, but it lacks iron, folic acid, and other nutrients babies need. Homemade evaporated milk formulas usually also lack iron and vitamin C.

Most of the commercial formulas come in a ready-to-feed form; a liquid concentrate, to which water must be added; and powder, which also must be mixed with water. The ready-to-feed type is most convenient and eliminates any concern about water safety (if you were to mix it with water the baby wouldn't get enough calories), but it is also the most expensive. Liquid concentrate, which comes in 13-ounce cans, must be mixed with equal parts water. Powdered formula is mixed by measuring one scoop of powder for every 2 ounces of water; the measuring must be done carefully, following the manufacturer's directions. Contrary to popular belief, powders are not much less expensive than liquid concentrates, but they do keep longer on the shelf—an advantage when a baby is mostly breastfed.

You may need to reevaluate your baby's fluoride needs when you wean. Too much fluoride can cause spotting on a baby's teeth. If you plan to use tap water to mix concentrated formula, ask your baby's doctor or your local water department to tell you the proportion of fluoride in the

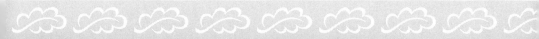

water. If your water contains 0.3 parts per million or more of fluoride and you have been giving fluoride supplements while breastfeeding, you should stop the supplements. If your water contains less fluoride than this, or if you are using only ready-to-feed formula or concentrate mixed with unfluoridated bottled water, your baby will need 0.25 milligrams of supplemental fluoride per day.

The cost of formula varies depending on the type (cow's milk, soy, or "predigested"), the form (ready-to-feed, liquid concentrate, or powder), and the brand, as well as the region of the country you live in and the store where you shop. The list that follows shows approximate monthly costs of supermarket-purchased formula for a baby who takes 32 ounces of formula per day (many babies take more). Costs of bottles, nipples, and other supplies—often including bottled water—must also be considered in weaning the young baby.

COW'S-MILK FORMULA
Ready-to-feed	$140–333
Liquid concentrate	125
Powder concentrate	100

SOY-MILK FORMULA
Ready-to-feed	171–333
Liquid concentrate	145
Powder concentrate	110

PREDIGESTED FORMULA
Ready-to-feed	240
Liquid concentrate	234
Powder concentrate	200

If you have a low family income, you might investigate whether you qualify for the WIC (Women, Infants, and Children) Supplemental Food Program, which is available in every state. WIC benefits for a qualifying family include food supplements if the mother is breastfeeding or formula coupons if the baby is bottle-fed (although not all formula brands are offered, and those that are offered are available only in iron-fortified forms). In addition, WIC nutritionists provide nutritional counseling during pregnancy and breastfeeding, and throughout infancy. You can find the phone number for a local WIC office in the governmental section of your phone directory, or get it from your city or county health department.

SELECTING BOTTLES AND NIPPLES

The best bottles are those that have accurate measuring indicators and are easy to clean. Plastic bottles are often inaccurate for measuring. Bottles that are molded into various shapes or split down the middle for self-feeding are almost impossible to clean adequately. Clear plastic bottles, when heated, may release harmful chemicals into milk. Although glass bottles may seem impractical, they don't break easily, they are easy to clean and sterilize, and they are generally the most accurate for measuring. Glass bottles can be hard to find in stores, but they can be ordered through the Internet. Some bottles require special nipples made by the same manufacturer.

Nipples are made of latex rubber or silicone. Silicone nipples are preferable, since rubber has a taste and a smell and deteriorates faster than silicone does. Rubber nipples are also harder to clean and should be washed by hand rather than in a dishwasher.

If you are considering using a disposable feeding system, keep a few things in mind. You can't sterilize formula using the disposable bags; the bags would break. With the pre-sterilized bags you can't accurately measure out water or formula concentrate; you have to mix the formula in a sterile container and then pour the mixture into the bags. Disposable feeding systems can save you work if you use ready-to-feed formula, which does not need to be sterilized or mixed, but you will still have to boil the nipples and caps. And don't be taken in by manufacturers' claims that a disposable feeding system is "most like breastfeeding" or that the "baby gets less air." All babies swallow some air as they suck; no bottle can prevent this (keeping the nipple of a regular bottle filled with liquid minimizes air swallowing just as well as a collapsible bag does). And a plastic bottle and rubber nipple are just that; the comparison to the breast is meant to play on your guilt feelings.

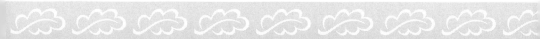

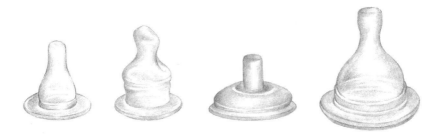

Four types of bottle nipples, from left to right: the longer conventional type, the flattened orthodontic type, the stubby type used in disposable feeding systems, and the broad-based European type, which must be used with the manufacturer's bottle.

GETTING YOUR BABY TO TAKE A BOTTLE

If your baby has had a bottle recently, she should have little trouble accepting one now. Babies who have willingly taken breast milk from a bottle, however, may object to the taste of formula at first. To make the transition easier, try offering breast milk mixed with a small amount of formula. Gradually increase the proportion of formula with each bottle you give the baby until she'll accept formula on its own.

A baby who has never had a bottle, or who has gone weeks with ut one, may strongly object to the whole idea. To get a baby used to the bottle, use only breast milk at first. Many mothers find that a longer, stiffer nipple or an orthodontic one (such as Nuk) is more readily accepted than the short, stubby kind common among disposable feeders. Some parents have had success with the Adiri Breastbottle Nurser, which is made of soft silicone to look and feel like a breast (this bottle can be ordered through the Internet). One technique that often works is to offer the bottle while walking, holding the baby facing outward. With one hand, cup her chin and hold the nipple in her mouth against her upper gum. If she has been crying, she will probably calm down and begin to mouth the nipple. Someone other than you may have more success in persuading the baby to accept the bottle at first.

Whether it's best to try the bottle when the baby is very hungry or only slightly hungry seems to vary among babies. Refusing to nurse a baby for hours in an attempt to force her to take a bottle is upsetting for everyone involved and rarely successful. Stop and try again later if either you or your baby gets too upset. Your patient persistence will pay off.

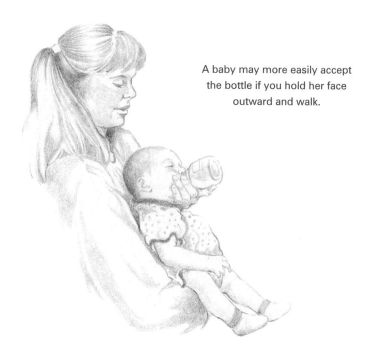

A baby may more easily accept the bottle if you hold her face outward and walk.

PREPARING FORMULA

If you have decided to wean your baby before he is three to four months old, it's best to use sterilizing techniques in preparing formula and bottles. Babies younger than about four months have very immature immune systems; that is, they are poorly able to fight off infection. Formula, unlike breast milk, provides no antibodies to protect an infant's health. The formula-fed baby is more susceptible to harmful bacteria, which can easily be transmitted from the hands of the feeder, rubber nipples, bottles, formula, water, and any of the food-preparation equipment or surfaces.

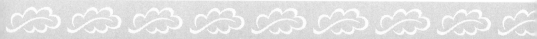

Many health-care providers have developed a casual attitude toward formula preparation: They feel that the work of sterilization is unnecessary. But many formula-fed infants do get gastrointestinal infections, and some of these babies must be hospitalized. Poor preparation and handling of bottles and formula, combined with a lack of antibodies from breast milk, may make many of these babies sick. Certainly it is best to err on the side of caution. Sterilizing equipment and formula has another advantage, too: You can prepare a whole day's supply of bottles and store them in the refrigerator, instead of preparing each bottle in the sometimes tense moments just before a feeding. Four sterilizing methods are described on pages 76–77.

If your baby is three to four months old, you can forego sterilization. With a clean sink and bottle brush, wash the bottles with hot, soapy water. Or use a dishwasher (with a water temperature of about 140 degrees F) on the full cycle, including pre-rinse. It's best to continue boiling the nipples; store them in a clean, dry, covered container. Mix formula in the bottle just before each feeding.

It is very important to follow the directions carefully when mixing liquid concentrate or powdered formula. Keep in mind that directions vary by brand, and companies change their instructions from time to time. Use the measuring equipment as well as the directions that come with the formula. Don't shake or tap the side of the measuring scoop; instead, level the powder off with the flat edge of a knife. When measuring water or liquid concentrate, use a clear glass measuring cup, and make sure levels are precise. As Ellyn Satter says in her excellent guide *Child of Mine: Feeding with Love and Good Sense* (2000), "When making up formula, don't get it close, GET IT RIGHT."

How to Sterilize Formula

A ny of these methods can be used with liquid concentrate. For powdered formula, some manufacturers recommend only the aseptic and single-bottle methods. With each method, you should begin by washing all of the supplies— bottles, nipples, caps, rings, can opener, and measuring and mixing utensils—in hot, soapy water.

For ready-to-feed formula, sterilize the equipment according to the aseptic method; put the nipples, rings, and caps on the bottles; and store the bottles for up to forty-eight hours. Just before each feeding, clean the can top with hot, soapy water, rinse the can, open it with a clean punch-type can opener, and pour the already sterile formula into the sterile bottle.

THE ASEPTIC METHOD

1. Place the clean bottles, nipples, caps, rings, punch-type can opener (for liquid formula), and measuring scoop in a sterilizer or a large pan with a rack or towel on the bottom. Cover everything with water, cover the pan, and bring the water to a boil. Boil for 5 minutes. Leave the equipment in the covered pan until the equipment is cool enough to handle.

2. In a kettle, bring fresh water just to a boil. Let it cool.

3. Wash and dry your hands, and then remove the equipment with tongs and place it on a clean towel. Be careful not to touch the insides of the bottles or nipples.

4. Wash the top of the formula can with hot, soapy water, and rinse.

5. If you're using liquid concentrate, shake the can well. Open the formula can with the can opener. Pour the correct amount of sterilized water into the bottles, and then add the liquid concentrate or powdered formula. Using the tongs, place the nipples upside down into the tops of the bottles. Add the rings and caps, and tighten them.

6. Shake the bottles. Store them in the refrigerator for use within 24 to 48 hours, as directed by the manufacturer.

THE TERMINAL STERILIZATION METHOD

1. Wash the top of the formula can with hot, soapy water, and rinse. If you're using liquid concentrate, shake the can well, and open it with a clean punch-type can opener.

2. Mix enough formula for a full day's use, stirring well.

3. Pour the prepared formula into the clean bottles. Place the nipples upside down on the bottles, and loosely put on the rings and caps.

4. Place the bottles in a sterilizer or on a rack or towel in a large pan with 3 inches of water. Cover the pan, and bring the water to a boil. Boil for 25 minutes. Turn off the heat, and leave the bottles in the covered pan for about an hour, until they are cool enough to handle.

5. Tighten the rings, and store the bottles in the refrigerator. Use them within 24 to 48 hours, as directed by the formula manufacturer.

SINGLE-BOTTLE METHOD I

1. Put the directed amount of cold water into each bottle.

2. Place the nipples upside down on the bottles, and loosely put on the rings and caps.

3. Place the bottles in a sterilizer or on a rack or towel in a large pan. Pour enough water into the pan to reach the level of water in the bottles.

4. Cover the pan, and bring the water to a boil. Boil for 25 minutes. Turn off the heat, and leave the bottles in the covered pan for about an hour, until they are cool enough to handle.

5. Tighten the caps, and store the bottles at room temperature for as long as 48 hours.

6. Just before each feeding, wash the top of the formula can with hot, soapy water, and rinse. If you're using liquid concentrate, shake the can well, and open it with a clean punch-type can opener. Add the specified amount of formula to the bottle, and shake well. Feed the baby promptly.

SINGLE-BOTTLE METHOD II

1. Put the clean bottles, nipples, caps, and rings into a sterilizer or on a rack or towel in a large pan. Cover everything with water, and bring the water to a boil. Boil for 5 minutes. Turn off the heat, and leave the bottles in the covered pan for about an hour, until they are cool enough to handle.

2. Wash and dry your hands, and then remove the equipment with tongs and place it on a clean towel. Be careful not to touch the insides of the bottles or nipples.

3. Assemble the bottles, nipples, rings, and caps. Store them at room temperature for up to 48 hours.

4. Shortly before feeding time, bring fresh water just to a boil. Let it cool.

5. Wash the top of the formula can with hot, soapy water, and rinse. Open the can with a clean punch-type can opener. Add the measured formula and sterile water to the sterile bottles. Shake well, and feed the baby promptly.

Overdiluting formula can slow a baby's growth by reducing the nutrients he receives. Underdiluting formula can burden a baby's kidneys
and digestive system and lead to dehydration. When you mix formula
for your baby, measure accurately!

EVALUATING YOUR WATER SUPPLY

Where your water comes from is important even if you're going to sterilize it. Municipal water districts are required by law to monitor for contaminants. Although most municipal water supplies meet federal
standards for safety, not all do. You may want to check with your water
department to find out whether the levels of bacteria, nitrates, heavy
metals, and sodium in your tap water are safe before you decide to use
the water for mixing formula. If you have private well water, have it
tested to be sure that the water is safe.

Municipal water supplies are chlorinated to lessen bacterial contamination, but tap water may still contain high levels of bacteria—a potential problem if you don't sterilize the water for your baby. The safety
of chlorine itself, for children or adults, is also doubtful; studies have associated chlorine in drinking water with higher levels of miscarriages
and of bladder and rectal cancer.

Nitrate levels of 10 milligrams or more per liter can react with the he-
moglobin in an infant's red blood cells to produce an anemic condition
commonly known as "blue baby" (methemoglobinemia). Such high nitrate levels, most commonly found in water supplies that originate in
farming areas, are increased by boiling the water.

Heavy metals are sometimes present in tap water. The most common
of these metals is lead. Lead poisoning, considered by public-health officials to be the number-one environmental health threat to children, can
lead to serious damage to the brain, nervous system, kidneys, and red
blood cells. Exposure to small amounts of lead can lower IQs, perhaps
permanently. In an estimated 20 percent of U.S. homes, the tap water
may contain dangerously high lead levels (15 micrograms or more per
liter). Lead can leach into water from lead pipes and connectors inside

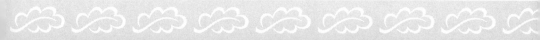

and outside the home; from bronze and brass faucets, which contain lead; and even from the solder used on copper pipes. Some babies have been poisoned with lead from the water used to mix their formula.

Lead levels in your drinking water are likely to be highest if your home has either lead pipes or copper pipes with lead solder. Although many people assume that only old plumbing carries the threat of lead contamination, tap water in a building less than five years old is particularly likely to have high lead levels, especially if the water is soft. This is because the solder in new pipes has not yet been coated with the mineral deposits that usually build up over time. Water that has remained in the pipes for several hours will have the highest lead levels.

The only way to be sure of the lead level in your tap water is to have the water tested in a laboratory. Your water or health department should be able to either perform the test or refer you to a laboratory that can.

Until you are sure your water is safe, buy bottled water, or at least let your cold water run for two minutes or more before using it to mix with formula (this flushing may be ineffective in a high-rise building). Never use hot water from the tap for mixing formula; it is likely to contain more lead. Boiling water does not eliminate lead, but actually increases the lead concentration.

High sodium levels in tap water can occur in coastal areas, where ocean water may mix with freshwater, and in homes with water-softening systems (although in newer systems the cold water often bypasses the water-softening process). When a baby is sick, feeding her a solution that is high in sodium can worsen her dehydration. The Environmental Protection Agency has set 20 milligrams per liter as the maximum safe level for sodium.

Buying bottled water is no guarantee of pure, safe water for your baby, although the bottled-water industry is subject to standards, which vary from state to state, similar to those governing municipal water departments. Water labeled as distilled, demineralized or de-ionized, or purified should be free of all contaminants. Spring water and water labeled "drinking" or "filtered" can be quite variable in quality, and may not be ideal for infants (one infant-food company is now selling bottled "spring water with fluoride," an expensive and unnecessary product). A properly maintained home reverse-osmosis system will also provide water that is free of contaminants.

While you're investigating the safety of your water, be sure to check on its fluoride content (see page 79).

STORING FORMULA AND WARMING BOTTLES

A can of formula can be safely stored, unopened, at room temperature so long as the expiration date on the can has not passed. Once the can has been opened, liquid concentrate or ready-to-feed formula can be stored, tightly covered, in the refrigerator for up to 48 hours. Powdered formula can be stored, covered, in a cool, dry place for as long as the manufacturer recommends—typically four weeks for cow's milk formula, three weeks for soy formula.

Refrigerate prepared formula or opened cans of liquid concentrate at 35 to 40 degrees F. Measure the refrigerator temperature with an accurate thermometer; if the temperature is higher than 40 degrees F, turn the thermostat down. Formula stored at higher than 40 degrees F must be considered contaminated after two hours, and thrown out.

If a bottle has formula left in it after you have fed your baby, the bottle can safely remain out at room temperature for up to an hour. After that, throw away any formula remaining in the bottle—it can become contaminated with bacteria from your baby's mouth. Immediately rinse the bottles, and squeeze cool water through the nipples, to make complete cleaning easier later on. Formula prepared and left out at room temperature for hours, perhaps in anticipation of night feedings, is unsafe.

Cold formula won't hurt a baby, but if you decide to warm your baby's bottles, do it just before feeding him. Don't warm bottles by letting them sit out at room temperature. Don't use a microwave oven, either; babies have been burned by formula overheated in a microwave, and microwaving can destroy some of the vitamins in formula. To heat a bottle, set it in a bowl of warm water or hold it under warm running tap water. Shake the bottle gently to distribute the warmth, and test a drop or two on your wrist (it should be lukewarm to the touch).

If your baby needs to be fed away from home, there are a few options for safe bottle feeding. If a bottle of prepared formula is well chilled, you can carry it with you for a couple of hours. Or you can take pre-sterilized bottles with the water in them, and mix in powdered formula just before

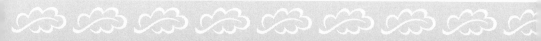

each feeding. Sterile disposable feeding bags make good containers for measured portions of powdered formula. Other options are to carry along a small cooler, and to purchase single ready-to-feed bottles (they are expensive).

DETERMINING HOW MUCH TO FEED

How much formula your baby takes is best determined by your baby. Most babies can be trusted to take as much as they need when they need it. After the first two weeks, many babies take as much as 32 ounces of breast milk or formula per day. Most young babies want three to six ounces per feeding and six to eight feedings per day. The actual amount of formula your baby drinks will also be influenced by her age, her growth pattern, her activity level, and other factors, such as illness. If you're worried about your baby's growth, your baby's doctor or nurse can show you just how it is progressing on your baby's growth chart.

You can figure that your baby will want 2.5 to 3 ounces of formula per day for each pound the baby weighs. For example, a baby who weighs 10 pounds requires 25 to 30 ounces of milk or formula per day.

Some formula-fed babies overfeed, to the point of obesity. Within an hour or two after a feeding, they may want to take several ounces more, or they may take tremendous amounts of formula every few hours. A baby who seems to overconsume formula—especially if she also has intestinal symptoms, such as spitting up, passing a lot of gas, an irritated rectal area, or frequent runny stools—may be intolerant of her formula, in which case a change should be considered. Some parents react to any fussiness by offering another full bottle. Babies do love to suck, and a bottle-fed baby may need something else to suck on. A pacifier or comfort nursing (even if you have little or no milk) may satisfy your baby and keep her from overconsuming formula.

BOTTLE FEEDING AS YOU HAVE BREASTFED

The tendency toward higher intellectual ability in breastfed children (see page 21) may originate partially in their frequent and prolonged contact with their mothers. The breast cannot be separate from the mother; her face, voice, and touch are always present during feedings, stimulating her baby to look at her, "talk" to her, touch her, and play with her. Bottle feeding, though never so physically intimate, can certainly be an opportunity for parent-child social interaction. Too often, parents ignore this opportunity. Because holding a baby for bottle feeding requires the use of two arms, it becomes an unpleasant chore for many parents. So they lay the baby down and, in one way or another, prop the bottle up. Bottle propping is dangerous: It can make a young baby choke and aspirate formula.

When a bottle-fed baby reaches about three months of age, he may be expected to feed himself. Although some parents see self-feeding as a developmental accomplishment, in encouraging it they deprive their babies of some very important contact and stimulation. Imagine what a baby misses out on when he spends his day sitting in an infant seat, feeding himself.

The bottle can become unhealthful in other ways, too. Babies often drop bottles and then put them back into their mouths, along with dirt and bacteria from the floor or the ground. Older babies and toddlers who carry around bottles all day, or go to sleep sucking at them, risk serious tooth decay.

Bottle-feed, then, much as you have breastfed. Hold your baby in your arms whenever you feed him, and have your mate and other caregivers do the same thing. Let the baby control his feeding as a breastfed baby does: Wait for him to open his mouth rather than pushing the nipple in yourself. Be patient when he pauses in sucking; don't stimulate him to suck continuously. Even if there is formula left in the bottle, let your baby stop drinking when he signals that he has had enough. Instead of putting your baby in a crib wide awake, let him drift peacefully off to sleep in your arms.

Regardless of your reason for weaning your baby early, you may have mixed feelings when breastfeeding comes to an end. If you expected to

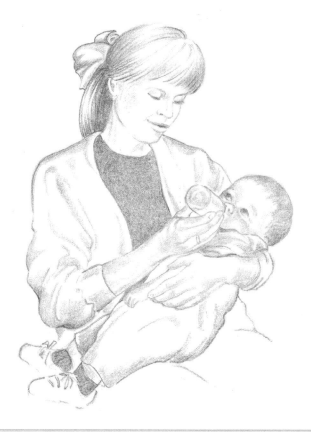

Bottle-feed as you have breastfed, with your baby in your arms. Remember that the bottle belongs to you, not your child.

nurse your baby longer, you may feel sad or even depressed. If you've struggled with breastfeeding difficulties and finally given up, you may feel relieved—but you may also feel that you've failed. Seeing other women nurse may stimulate strong feelings in you for some time to come.

Remember that, no matter how long you nursed your baby, he has benefited from breastfeeding. You gave your baby the best possible start in life, and you established a close bond that will last for the rest of your lives.

three

WEANING YOUR FOUR-
TO TWELVE-MONTH-OLD

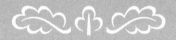

A
S WITH YOUNGER BABIES, there are many reasons that women consider weaning babies over four months old. Perhaps you have been struggling with sore nipples, biting episodes, or a baby who seems to be growing less interested in nursing. You may be facing going back to work, or maybe you're pregnant again. Several situations that may be causing you to consider weaning (such as breast infections, upcoming separations, or your need to take medications) are discussed in Chapter 2, "Weaning Before Four Months." Perhaps you want to get back into shape by dieting. Or maybe you, your family, or your friends simply think that your baby is "old enough" to stop nursing.

Whatever your situation, it is important that you thoroughly consider your circumstances and carefully measure the advantages of weaning against the value of breastfeeding to you and, most important, to your baby. Formula feeding is not without its own costs, hassles, and risks (see "The Hazards of Formula Feeding" in Chapter 1, pages 19-24). Weaning an older baby, while fairly easy to accomplish, can be difficult to reverse.

> The American Academy of Pediatrics recommends that babies be breastfed throughout their first year, and given no other foods besides breast milk during the first six months.

Nursing Your Older Baby

Although difficulties with breastfeeding can arise at any time, nursing the older baby is usually easy, convenient, and rewarding. Most nursing mothers of older babies appreciate the health benefits that breast milk provides infants, and also the emotional closeness that develops between mother and baby. Nursing at this age comforts during sickness and soothes hurts. Nursing also helps a tired baby fall quickly and quietly off to sleep.

Throughout the entire first year of life and beyond, breastfeeding provides babies with the best possible nourishment and the best defense against infection. Even babies who nurse just a few times a day tend to be much healthier than those who do not breastfeed at all. Babies weaned at the end of the first year tend to be healthier in the second year than babies weaned earlier (Gulick 1986).

When a mother weans her baby before he is a year old, she must provide an iron-fortified infant formula, the best substitute for breast milk. The introduction of solid foods to a baby's diet does not eliminate his need for milk. In fact, until he takes three meals of table food plus snacks each day, usually at around eight to ten months, he should continue to have a milk feeding before he eats his solids.

Some babies stop nursing voluntarily at about nine to twelve months of age. Firstborn children, some say, have more of a tendency to wean on their own in the first year. This may be because first-time mothers, fascinated by each developmental milestone, tend to encourage "grown-up" behavior by offering their babies the breast less often. According to T. Berry Brazelton (1983), many infants at five months, seven months, and nine to twelve months show less interest in breastfeeding because they are busy developing new abilities, such as crawling, standing, and walking. Perhaps some mothers interpret this temporary decline in interest as their babies' desire to wean. In cases like this, however, it is the mother who weans, not the baby.

When a baby is still nursing often and enthusiastically at the end of his first year, he will probably want to continue nursing throughout the second year and beyond.

According to Ruth Lawrence, a pediatrician and lactation expert, children rarely initiate weaning between ages one and four. For this reason friends may tell you to initiate weaning yourself by your baby's first birthday if you have definite feelings against nursing a three-year-old. You may fear that, if you wait, you will have a major struggle convincing your child to stop nursing in the months to follow. That toddlers seldom initiate weaning, however, doesn't mean they always fight it. If you find yourself still happily nursing at your baby's first birthday, keep in mind that the next three years will probably bring several opportune times to wean, by any of numerous techniques.

Difficulties that you may have encountered while nursing your older baby—tiredness after a return to work or school, frequent night nursing, or being bitten—may make you wonder if the bottle wouldn't make things easier somehow. If nursing your baby is routine and mostly pleasurable, you may still have mixed feelings about continuing.

Even the happiest nursing mother sometimes has ambivalent feelings about nursing. The wants and needs of your child will undoubtedly collide with your own desires from time to time, not only while you're nursing but throughout your parenting years. Although ambivalence may be an irritating feeling, it does not necessarily mean you should wean. However long you choose to nurse, it helps to appreciate that breastfeeding, like mothering in general, has its ups and downs.

If you have been struggling with some difficulty, weaning to formula may seem to be the best solution. Maybe it is, but then again maybe it isn't. The section that follows may help you decide whether weaning is the best way to resolve your problem.

Possible Reasons to Wean Your Older Baby

TOO OLD TO NURSE?

During your pregnancy you may have assumed you would breastfeed for a certain time period—perhaps the length of time friends or relatives nursed, or the period in which you believed breast milk would be valuable to a baby. Maybe you thought babies needed breast milk only until they started eating solid foods. Even if you believe otherwise now, you may feel compelled to follow through with your plans.

Or maybe you'd like to continue nursing, but other people think your baby is simply "too old." Family members and friends who encouraged you in the early days of nursing may no longer be supportive. They may make mildly disapproving comments or pretend to ignore that you're still nursing. This happens to many nursing mothers as their babies get older. Although the comments about nursing may not be overtly critical, they get across the message that nursing should stop. Most women are very vulnerable to others' opinions about their mothering.

So when does a baby no longer need the breast? In terms of immunological maturity, twelve-month-olds are just reaching 60 percent of adult capability for fighting infection. In terms of emotional maturity, children stop needing the security of the breast at widely varying ages. Whereas some babies happily wean at nine months, others need the comfort of the breast for much longer. But our society is intolerant of children's natural dependencies. We rush babies and young children toward independence. Perhaps we fear that by meeting a baby's needs we are spoiling her or keeping her from growing up.

Meeting a baby's needs through breastfeeding actually helps a baby become more independent. Having the security of the breast bolsters a baby's confidence to explore outside her mother's arms. At any time her bravery is shaken, she knows she can return to the comfort of her mother's breast.

Independence grows out of a child's faith that her source of security will always be there when she needs it.

Knowing all this, you may still have trouble dealing with the disapproval of friends and family members. Families in particular can wield tremendous influence over a nursing relationship; we know of several young mothers whose own mothers refused to baby-sit until the grandchild was weaned. You may be able to deal with criticism from others by either ignoring it or confronting it. Or you may choose to withdraw from those who are critical, and find new friends who believe in nursing older babies; a mother-to-mother support group such as La Leche League is one place to do this. Finally, you might simply keep your nursing secret from those who disapprove.

None of these strategies may work, though, if your mate is among your critics. In this case you may ultimately be too uncomfortable to continue nursing. Perhaps you can persuade him to read "The Hazards of Formula Feeding" in Chapter 1 (pages 19-24), or show him the chart on the cost of formula on page 71. And, if your baby is waking at night for feedings, tell your mate that if you wean he can take over night duty.

SHARP TEETH AND BITING

Between ages four months and one year, a baby starts cutting teeth. Occasionally a mother's nipples are irritated by her baby's new top teeth during nursing. This seems to happen most commonly when the top teeth next to the front ones come in first. When new teeth erupt, they are very thin and sharp; they have to be in order to push through the gums. New teeth become much thicker and less irritating after a few weeks. Until this happens, try varying your baby's position at the breast and giving him some teething toys to help wear down the sharp tooth edges.

Mothers often fear that their babies will start biting once teeth appear. This occasionally happens, but it is usually because other areas of the gums are sore and not because the baby wants to try out his new teeth. A baby who bites usually does so just before new teeth come in. He can't bite while he is sucking, because then his tongue covers his lower gum. But when he stops sucking, he can pull back his tongue and bite down.

If you have been bitten, keep a few things in mind. Biting usually occurs at the end of a feeding, or any time the baby is not really interested in nursing. During teething, keep your nursings all-business and brief, ending them as soon as your baby slows down in his sucking and swallowing. Some mothers notice that their babies get playful looks on their faces just before biting. If you notice such a look, end the feeding.

If you miss your baby's cues and get bitten, say "NO!" and end the feeding. Do not nurse him again for at least a half-hour, or until you feel certain he is hungry. If you react this way consistently, the biting will probably end within a few days, as suddenly as it began. It is unnecessary and inappropriate to hit a baby or bite him back.

Once in a great while a mother will be bitten hard enough that the skin behind the nipple is broken. If this happens to you, be sure to keep the area clean; you can dribble a little hydrogen peroxide on the cut after nursing. Nursing from the breast may be too painful, though; in this case, express your milk until the injury heals. If the skin remains broken for several days, you may need an oral antibiotic for healing to occur.

Sometimes a mother thinks a sore nipple must be the result of a bite even though she can't remember being bitten. In such a case the pain and the appearance of the nipple usually suggest another cause, most often thrush or a plug in the nipple opening (see "Sore Nipples," the next section, and pages 28-33).

SORE NIPPLES

Sore nipples can occur for several reasons after the early months of breastfeeding. The baby's position during nursing is usually not the cause of the problem.

Most often, nipple irritation after the early weeks is caused by thrush or yeast. Although yeast infections occasionally happen for unknown reasons, frequently they occur within a few weeks after a course of antibiotics is taken by either mother or baby. The nipples are typically pink or red; the skin of the nipple and areola can be rashy, peeling, or even cracked. The nipples typically burn, and there may also be pain inside the breast. The baby may or may not have the characteristic white patches of thrush in her mouth, and may or may not have a yeast diaper rash. Even if the baby shows no obvious signs of oral thrush, you may have to treat her as well as your nipples to eliminate the infection. For advice on treating thrush, see "Sore Nipples" in Chapter 2 (pages 28-33).

A plugged nipple opening is another possible cause of nipple pain. The breast may hurt behind the nipple, too, and may not empty in this area with nursing. The nipple with a plugged opening looks normal in color, but a white spot can be seen on the nipple tip, particularly right after the baby comes off the breast. For suggestions on treatment, see "Plugged Ducts" in Chapter 2 (pages 49–51).

A mother's nipples may also feel tender for several days between the time of ovulation and the onset of menstruation, and in early pregnancy. This soreness is not associated with any visible signs, such as redness or another abnormality on the nipple or areola. Mid-cycle nipple tenderness may occur prior to only some menstrual periods, or it may occur monthly; it disappears just as a woman's period begins. If your periods haven't resumed yet, such tenderness may indicate that they will very soon. If it continues and your period doesn't come, the tenderness may indicate that you're pregnant. A mild pain reliever and anti-inflammatory such as ibuprofen may help reduce pain during nursing, and is safe to take unless you're pregnant.

Nipple problems other than the common ones just described can also occur after the early months of breastfeeding. The nipple and surrounding area, like other areas of skin, are subject to irritation, inflammation, and infection. A visit with a lactation professional or a dermatologist may help in diagnosing and ending the problem.

RETURNING TO WORK

If you are returning to work, see the discussion on this topic in Chapter 2 (pages 51–55). Several additional considerations apply when you're facing regular separations from an older baby.

Although some mothers assume they must wean before going back to work, many mothers of older babies find that continuing to nurse provides many advantages. Combining nursing and working is usually easier with an older baby than with a very young one.

By the time a baby reaches four months to a year, his mother's milk production is generally well established, and he may be taking solid foods in addition to breast milk. Continuing to breastfeed, even if you also feed formula part time, can help your baby stay healthier, which means you may miss fewer days of work. Besides, leaving your baby is difficult enough for both of you; weaning would be an added loss. When you continue to nurse, each homecoming is a loving reunion.

You may still have doubts about continuing to breastfeed, though, when you imagine yourself expressing milk at work. If your baby is still reliant on milk every two to three hours, and is not taking much in the way of solids, you will need to decide whether you want to express milk while you're away. Take into consideration how many hours you'll be gone. Working part time—say, no more than twenty-four hours per week—without expressing will have much less effect on your milk supply than working full time without expressing. You can best maintain your milk supply by spreading out your hours—for instance, by working four hours or fewer per day, or by working every other day, with extra nursings while you are with your baby. Regardless of how many hours you work, if you can express even once while away you will be more likely to maintain your supply. Expressing two or three times if you are gone eight to nine hours will not only help maintain your supply but will also eliminate the need for much formula.

The type of breast pump you choose makes all the difference in the ease of expressing milk while you are away. Be sure to read "Returning to Work" in Chapter 2 for a complete discussion of breast pumps.

If you are working full time or nearly so, and are unable or unwilling to express milk, you will need to substitute formula for missed nursings. Because your milk supply will lessen, you may also need to offer formula at some feedings on your days off. Your baby may be quite happy to continue nursing before and after work and in the night, if he still wakes, or he may come to refuse the breast if the milk takes too long to let down or the supply becomes too low (be sure to distinguish between refusal to nurse because of low milk production and the normal distractibility that the older baby often exhibits when there is something else going on around him). Although a baby may wean when the milk supply drops off, he certainly will have benefited from the breast milk he has received up to that point.

A baby who is eight months old or older, and who is well established on solid foods, may be easiest to nurse part time. Although milk production may decline when feedings are missed and the breasts are not emptied during work hours, the baby may be very happy to nurse in the morning, at night, and during your days off. You may be able to avoid bottle feeding altogether if your baby can get a sufficient amount of formula from a cup at mealtimes.

To maintain your milk production while you are working—

◆ Nurse frequently when you and your baby are together. This is especially important if you don't express milk at work.

◆ Nurse once or twice in the morning before work, and as soon as possible upon returning to your baby.

◆ Wake your baby to nurse just before you go to bed if he sleeps through most of the night.

Sleeping with your baby can encourage night nursing and can make it easy to nurse often without disrupting your sleep much.

NEGLECTED SIBLINGS

If you have an older child, you're probably acutely aware of how neglected she has felt during the past few months. It is nature's intent that most of your attention be focused on your new baby, but knowing this may not relieve your guilt feelings. Although you might like to spend more time with your older child, it may seem as if every time you start to play or read with her the baby wants to nurse, and of course the baby comes first. Your older child, purposely or not, may distract the baby from nursing or wake him just after you've gotten him to sleep, or get into mischief elsewhere in the house while you're nursing. There may be times when your patience runs thin, and after you lose your temper you may feel even more guilty than before. Will weaning allow you to divide your attention more fairly among your children?

Whether you wean or not, your older child will never again get the attention of an only child. After weaning you'll still spend a lot of time diapering, soothing, and getting the baby to sleep, as well as preparing and feeding bottles. But you can nurse the baby without totally shutting out your older child.

There are several things you can try in order to create more calm:

◆ Forewarn your older child before you plan to nurse the baby, so you can both focus on getting settled.

◆ Sit on the floor to nurse so you can stay involved in your older child's activities.

◆ Prepare a quiet activity that your child can manage alone in your presence. Some mothers have found that putting aside special toys, puzzles, or crayons and paper just for these times can create ten or twenty minutes of quiet.

◆ Prepare a small meal or snack for both you and your older child to enjoy while you nurse the baby.

◆ Read to your older child while you nurse, if this doesn't distract the baby too much.

◆ Go outside into the yard or to a park, if weather permits, so your older child can have fun while you nurse in peace.

◆ Allow your older child to lie quietly beside you on the bed while you nurse the baby at naptime. With any luck both children may go to sleep.

Try to arrange for some special time alone with your older child. Perhaps the two of you can go off together for a few hours of fun. Encourage your mate or other adults to spend time with your older child as well.

DISTRACTIBILITY AND NURSING STRIKES

You may notice that at around four to five months your baby becomes easily distracted during nursing. At any new, sudden, or interesting sight or sound, she pulls away from the breast to look around. This doesn't mean she wants to wean. After several weeks she will no longer have to interrupt herself to check out what's going on around her; she'll just turn her head with the nipple still in her mouth. In the meantime, you may find that nursing in a quiet or semi-darkened room helps your baby complete her feedings.

Sometimes babies actually refuse to nurse for a while. Although "nursing strikes" can occur at any time, they most often happen in the second half of a baby's first year. A nursing strike is usually distinguished from weaning by its suddenness. A few babies wean themselves between eight and twelve months, but they usually do so gradually.

Reasons for a nursing strike vary. They include teething, a cold, an ear infection, a painful sore in the mouth, or a change in the taste of the milk. They sometimes happen after a prolonged separation between a baby and her mother, or after a baby has bitten her mother and has been frightened by the response. Sometimes when a baby has grown used to the rapid flow of milk from a bottle, her refusal to nurse is a response to her mother's dwindling milk supply (in this case the baby's refusal, however sudden, is self-weaning). Some authorities believe a nursing strike may precede a baby's mastery of a major motor skill, such as crawling, standing, or walking.

Although some mothers decide to turn a nursing strike into final weaning, in most cases the baby can be coaxed to resume nursing. Strikes typically last several hours to a few days, but may go on for as long as two weeks. During the time that your baby is reluctant to nurse, try a change in position, or nurse in a quiet, darkened room. Try offering the breast whenever your baby is sleepy. For as long as she refuses to nurse, express your milk frequently throughout the day if you wish to maintain or rebuild your supply. Offer the breast milk in a cup rather than a bottle. If your baby's refusal persists for longer than a couple of days, have her examined to rule out an ear infection or other physical problem.

WANTING TO GET BACK INTO SHAPE

If you longed during pregnancy to have your old body back, you may feel disappointed or even resentful that it still hasn't returned. Many women dislike the size and shape of their postpartum bodies. It can be difficult to accept that the body you now see is the normal outcome of pregnancy. You may be anxious to begin serious dieting, exercising, or both.

Maybe you've heard that other women have lost weight simply by weaning. Many women do lose weight when they stop breastfeeding, but mostly this is the weight of milk in the breasts. The thighs, buttocks, and abdomen aren't necessarily affected.

Because breastfeeding mothers burn a lot of calories in the production of milk, most gradually lose extra pounds without a weight-loss diet. Certainly women who breastfeed tend to lose more weight in the first year after birth than those who bottle-feed—especially between three and six months postpartum, when milk production is highest. And the more often a woman breastfeeds, the more rapidly she tends to lose weight.

If you're not losing weight effortlessly, though, you can diet while nursing. We don't recommend crash or fad diets because they usually are unhealthful and rarely produce long-lasting results. Losing weight too rapidly could also release pesticides and other toxins from your body into your milk. But simply limiting calories so that you lose one to two pounds a week should not harm either your baby or your milk.

Some women feel and look fat when they really just have loose abdominal muscles. Abdominal strengthening exercises can help improve your appearance and posture. Elizabeth Noble's *Essential Exercises for the Childbearing Year* (2003) is a good guide for developing strength and flexibility.

Exercising promotes not only muscular firmness, weight control, and vitality, but milk production as well. A supportive bra provides comfort during vigorous exercise. Exercise bras, which provide very good support, can be pulled up for nursing.

O ne study (Lonnerdal et al. 1990) found that mothers who exercised not only lost weight as fast as or faster than non-exercising mothers (while eating more), they also made more milk.

You can start getting more exercise in any of a number of ways. You can join a class or a health club; many exercise centers even offer child care. If you take a mother-baby exercise class, you won't need child care at all. If you'd like to walk or run with the baby or the whole family, you'll find plenty of good equipment available, such as high-quality baby backpacks and jogging strollers.

FATIGUE AND INTERRUPTED SLEEP

One reason you may be considering weaning is plain old tiredness. You may feel as tired in the morning as when you went to sleep the night before, or you may simply lack energy to accomplish much during the day. You may wonder if nursing isn't to blame, and if switching to the bottle wouldn't make life easier.

Chances are your baby isn't sleeping through the night. He may in fact be waking more at night and napping less during the day than he did in the first few months. Perhaps adding to your fatigue are increased activities outside the home, or even a marginal diet.

"Oh, for just one night's uninterrupted sleep!" may be your bleary-eyed lament. You may have thought that, when your baby reached this age and, perhaps, started taking solid food, his nighttime wakings would diminish. You probably even know someone whose baby "sleeps through the night." It is a myth, however, that babies should sleep all night long without waking. When health professionals talk about sleeping through the night, they are referring to a six-hour stretch. Although some babies sleep a six-hour stretch by the age of six months, it is unreasonable to expect most babies to sleep even this long. At about four months of age, in fact, many babies who were sleeping long stretches begin waking more frequently.

Parents in our society have been led to believe that something is wrong when their babies don't sleep through the night. A parent may search for the reason that her child wakes. Teething, illness, hunger, thirst, digestive problems, wet diapers, chilling or overheating, superior intelligence, upcoming developmental milestones, and separation anxiety are only some of the explanations health professionals give to parents about why their babies continue waking at night.

As you may suspect, breastfed babies are less likely than bottle-fed babies to sleep through the night by the second half of the first year. Chances are your friend's sleeping baby is already weaned, or was never nursed at all. One study found that whereas weaned babies slept a median of nine to ten hours at a stretch at every age after four months, nursing babies slept in bouts of four to seven hours up to the end of the second year (Elias et al. 1986).

Not only do breastfed babies sleep in shorter bouts than do those who are bottle-fed, but they also sleep less overall. In the Elias study, weaned babies slept a median of thirteen to fourteen hours daily throughout the first two years, but nursing babies gradually lessened their total hours of sleep from a median of fourteen to a median of eleven hours.

There may be a number of reasons why bottle-fed babies sleep in longer stretches than do breastfed babies. Marsha Walker (1993b), a lactation consultant, points out that babies formula-fed from birth have poor "vagal nerve tone"; that is, their autonomic nervous systems are measurably disordered. This makes them sleepier and less alert than breastfed newborns. Poor vagal tone in a newborn, moreover, is related to inferior motor and mental development for at least two years after birth.

Babies who are weaned after several months of breastfeeding may start sleeping through the night for other reasons. They certainly have waking episodes, as we all do, but these children fall back into deep sleep without any intervention from parents. Most have probably learned to go back to sleep alone—sometimes by sucking a thumb, occasionally with a sophisticated method such as scheduled awakenings (whereby a parent arouses a child in time to prevent spontaneous awakenings, until both spontaneous and scheduled awakenings are gradually eliminated), but most often through parents' simple refusal to respond to the babies' cries. Generally, the parents' desire for separation has overcome the baby's natural urge for closeness.

No one knows for sure why weaned children sleep more overall than those who are still nursing. We think children often nurse during light sleep; they release the nipple when they fall into deep sleep. This may be why a child who was obviously tired will, instead of falling asleep after a long nursing, sit up, seeming completely refreshed.

If nursing in a light-sleep state were counted as sleep, the average total hours of sleep might not vary at all between nursing and weaned children.

Not only do parents try hard to identify a reason for night waking, but many also spend a considerable amount of energy trying to end it. Feeding solids late in the evening, giving pain relievers or cold remedies (even when the baby isn't sick or in pain), trying to keep the baby from falling asleep while at the breast, consulting health-care providers, and trying different tactics in the middle of the night rarely work.

This is not to say that your baby shouldn't be examined if you suspect a physical discomfort. He may have an ear infection (especially if he's had a runny nose in the past couple of weeks), or he may be bothered at night by teeth working their way in. Some babies who are frequently distracted during daytime nursings may wake at night out of hunger.

Substituting pacifiers, bottles, and other comfort objects in the night is not likely to get you a full night's sleep, either. Many parents find themselves getting up at night to search for these items when their babies wake up crying, having lost them. And unless a bottle is filled with water, a baby risks developing dental caries when he drinks from one at bedtime and during the night.

If you are determined to make your baby sleep through the night, the only way you're likely to accomplish this is to let him cry it out for a few nights or more. There are a few books on this topic, perhaps the best known being Richard Ferber's *Solve Your Child's Sleep Problems: The Complete Practical Guide for Parents* (2006). The basic premise of these books is that the persistent night waker should and can be trained to sleep through the night. This means not picking up the child during the night when he wakes, but letting him cry himself back to sleep, until he learns that his crying is fruitless. Although this may seem drastic, many parents report that it has worked for them.

A gentler approach can be found in Elizabeth Pantley's *The No-Cry Sleep Solution* (2002). A mother of four, Pantley offers a six-step method for teaching babies to sleep all night. According to Pantley, 92 percent of parents who have used this method have succeeded at getting their babies to sleep through the night within two months, and slightly more than 50 percent have succeeded within three weeks.

The no-cry method involves early and long naps during the day, before-bed routines, early bedtimes, and, most important, a quick response when the baby wakes at night. When the baby cries, you immediately nurse her back to sleep. As time goes on, she becomes able to go back to sleep sooner, with fewer interventions. If the baby sleeps in her own crib, you gradually shorten her time at the breast until you can put her back when she is drowsy but not yet asleep. This takes patience; during the first several days, the baby may fully waken on being laid in the crib, and you may have to pick her up and nurse her again. When the baby can fall back to sleep after a short nursing, the next step is to comfort the baby without picking her up, by using a key word and patting her back. Eventually, the baby can be settled with just a word.

If either of these methods seems too extreme, or if neither works for you, you might consider doing what mothers of nursing children all over the world have done for millennia to make night waking less disruptive: Sleep with your baby. As James J. McKenna (1993) has written, "Infants sleeping for long periods in social isolation from parents constitutes an extremely recent cultural experiment, the biological and psychological consequences of which have never been evaluated." Still, you may have concerns and fears about sharing your bed with your baby. Contrary to popular belief, a baby will not be smothered by the covers or by a parent turning over. Parents who have tried this arrangement have found that after a few nights they adjust to the new sleeping companion, and his presence does not disrupt their sleep as much as did waking to his cries, getting out of bed, tending to him, and coming back to bed again. If taking a baby into bed puts a damper on the parents' sexual activity, couples who have adopted this approach seldom complain about a lack of sex. Parents say how much they enjoy watching their baby sleep, cuddling his warm little body, and waking up with him in the morning. Since the baby has easy access to the breast, he cries less at night. Neither the mother nor the baby needs to waken completely, and Dad needn't waken at all.

Families have come up with many inventive approaches to make the "family bed" more comfortable, safe, and convenient. You might invest in a larger mattress, build a platform for mattresses placed side by side, or simply put the mattress on the floor. So your mattress stays dry, get a waterproof mattress pad; so you stay dry, double-diaper the baby or consider using disposables at bedtime (if you aren't using them already). This will eliminate most nighttime diaper changes, too. When you must get up, a low-wattage night-light can make things easier.

If you have doubts about this "family bed" approach to nighttime parenting, you might still try it for a couple of weeks before dismissing the idea. You can find more detailed information on bed sharing in Deborah Jackson's *Three in a Bed* (1999) and Jay Gordon and Maria Goodavage's *Good Nights: The Happy Parents' Guide to the Family Bed* (2002). If you're still feeling worn out after you've found some way to get more sleep at night, you might examine your diet. Some breastfeeding professionals believe that some lactating women are vulnerable to fatigue because of vitamin B deficiencies. Although in such a case the baby will generally grow well and get the nutrients he needs from his mother's milk, she may suffer from low energy levels. Be sure you are eating plenty of whole grains, which are rich in B vitamins.

You might also consider supplementing your diet with brewer's yeast, an especially potent source of B vitamins that is thought to be more effective and faster-acting than B-complex vitamin pills. Available in any health-food store, brewer's yeast can be taken in tablet form or as a powder to be mixed with juice or milk. Start with the daily dose recommended on the label, and slowly increase the amount as needed to two to four times the daily recommendation. You can take brewer's yeast in this amount as long as you are nursing. Just don't increase the amount too quickly, or both you and your baby could get diarrhea.

ANOTHER PREGNANCY

Maybe you want to wean so you can get pregnant again. Perhaps a desire to have children closely spaced, previous difficulty in getting pregnant, or concern about your ticking "biological clock" has made you want another pregnancy soon after the last. Or maybe you already are pregnant, and you want to wean or think you must wean because of this.

If you are planning another pregnancy, you should know that unless your periods have returned chances are slim that you are fertile and able to conceive. Worldwide, most nursing mothers experience a one- to two-year respite from menstruation after each birth. Among U.S. nursing women, the resumption of periods is generally sooner, probably because we tend to nurse less frequently than other women. Adding supplemental foods to a baby's diet doesn't hasten the return of fertility unless the frequency of suckling and length of suckling time are reduced.

If you are having regular periods, and you are having symptoms of ovulation (mid-cycle stringy mucus or basal body temperature changes), continuing to nurse will not hurt your chance of getting pregnant. Of course, even if you are fertile you have no guarantee of conceiving. The average couple has only a 20 percent chance of conception each month with unprotected mid-cycle intercourse.

If your period has yet to return, you might consider reducing the frequency of nursings for several weeks to see if this will stimulate menstruation. If your baby is nursing at night, you might consider weaning during sleeping hours. If your baby already sleeps a long stretch at night, cutting back on nursing during the day and evening may help. Six to eight weeks should be a sufficient amount of time to see if cutting back on nursing brings on your period. If you completely wean, your period should return within six weeks. If after eight weeks it has not, you might want to consult your doctor.

Although many people, including some health professionals, frown on breastfeeding during pregnancy, there is no reason you cannot continue nursing your baby when you find out another is on the way. Nursing won't lead to a miscarriage or a malnourished newborn even if you feel too queasy during the early weeks of pregnancy to eat much.

Pregnancy often causes a decrease in milk supply during the early weeks and months, and some time in the second half of pregnancy the breasts revert to producing colostrum for the newborn. If your baby is much younger than a year, and you notice your milk supply declining, you may need to supplement with formula. Some nursing babies and toddlers wean themselves at some point during their mothers' pregnancies. Others do not seem to mind the changes in the milk, and show no signs of wanting to give up nursing.

Many women who nurse while pregnant experience tender breasts and sore nipples. These are due to the hormonal changes of pregnancy. Many women also feel especially tired at first—this again is a normal response to pregnancy. Plenty of rest can help combat fatigue, especially in the first trimester.

Although weaning won't make you feel any less tired, if you are suffering with sore nipples it certainly will put an end to painful nursing. Nipple tenderness due to pregnancy usually fades as the pregnancy progresses, but, while the tenderness lasts, there is no known cure for it except weaning. To determine whether your nipples are tender for another reason, see pages 90-91.

Some pregnant mothers notice uterine contractions while nursing. No studies have shown that such contractions lead to premature labor, but if you have had a previous premature labor you should discuss this possibility with your doctor.

If you do want to wean and your child is younger than a year, it may be best to delay weaning at least until she is regularly eating solid foods and drinking from a cup.

In the second and third trimesters of pregnancy, an excellent diet is essential for the nursing mother.

THE BABY WHO ISN'T EATING WELL

At some time between ages four and seven months babies become developmentally ready for solid foods, and begin to benefit from them nutritionally. Between eight and ten months babies should be offered a wide variety of table foods that together make up a nutritious diet. At this age a baby should also be learning to drink from a cup.

If your baby is reluctant to take solids but is an avid nurser, you may be somewhat anxious about whether he is eating a sufficient amount of food. You may wonder if you should wean him to force him into taking solids. More detailed guidelines on introducing solid foods for a healthful diet can be found under "How to Wean Your Older Baby" (page 106). Reading that section will give you reasonable expectations of what and how much your baby should be eating.

When feeding solids to your baby, keep several rules in mind:

◆ Be patient; wait until he is ready for each spoonful. Let your baby set the pace of feeding. If he wants to examine his food before deciding whether to eat it, let him.

◆ As soon as your baby wants to feed himself with fingers or spoon, let him.

◆ When he tells you he's had enough, either by turning his head away, keeping his mouth shut, or trying to get out of his chair, stop feeding him.

◆ In general, allow him to be in control of the feeding.

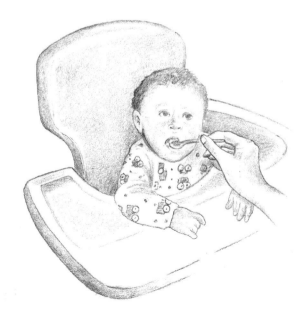

Until your baby is about eight to ten months old, milk is still the most important food in his diet. Offer solid foods only after nursing him. If he is reluctant to eat, cutting out nursing would only deprive him of the food he needs most—milk.

At around eight to ten months of age, most babies begin to eat more, until soon they are getting most of their calories from table food. At this age offer food about five times a day (three meals and two snacks). Nursing at this time continues to be important for early-morning feedings, snacks, naps, bedtime, and general soothing and comforting. To encourage the baby to take more solid foods, nursing is best delayed until after meals.

If your baby is taking few solids at best, try not to worry. Probably the biggest mistake parents can make in this situation is trying to force, trick, or pressure a baby into eating. These tactics often make a baby more reluctant to accept food. Food battles can escalate even more during the toddler period.

> Offer a wide variety of foods at mealtimes, keep a pleasant social atmosphere at the table, assist the baby in getting started, and let him stay in control of how much, if any, he eats.

Babies normally grow more slowly in the second six months after birth than they do in the first. For breastfed babies this is even more true than for formula-fed babies. A baby's weight gain during this period depends on genetic potential, activity level, and frequency and severity of illness as well as caloric intake. If your baby slows significantly in her weight gain or if her growth curve on a doctor's chart unexpectedly drops, you may feel pressure to make drastic changes. Keep in mind that your doctor is probably using a chart developed for formula-fed babies; although growth charts for breastfed babies are now available, they are not yet used by most health-care providers. Certainly it is important to make sure that a physical problem is not causing a baby to gain poorly. If you conclude that your baby, while otherwise healthy, is getting too little nourishment, there are certain things you can do.

The four- to seven-month-old who is gaining weight poorly will benefit from more milk and, if she seems ready, the addition of solid foods.

Replacing breast milk with formula would make no sense, since breast milk and formula have the same caloric value. You may be able to increase your breast-milk production by increasing the number of daily feedings to seven or eight. If this is not possible, or if you are already nursing this often, try offering some formula after breastfeeding—either an ounce or two several times a day or a larger amount after breastfeeding at bedtime. Iron-fortified infant cereal, mixed with breast milk or formula and offered after breastfeeding, can also provide more calories.

Even though you may be very anxious because your baby isn't gaining weight, be careful not to pressure her about food. She should have the right to determine when she's had enough. Your job is to offer milk and food periodically throughout the day in a supportive and patient manner.

The eight- to twelve-month-old who is gaining too little weight should be offered a wide variety of table foods, along with milk or formula from a cup at each mealtime and snack time. To maximize the baby's appetite at mealtimes, nursing or bottles are best delayed until after meals. Once again, let the baby take charge of what and how much she eats and drinks.

More detailed advice on feeding solids to the older baby can be found later in this chapter, on pages 114-18. A nutritionist can provide additional guidance.

How to Wean Your Older Baby

If you are clear in your desire to stop nursing, there are many things to consider: how quickly to proceed, what infant formula to wean to, how to get your baby to accept a bottle, whether to wean to a cup, how to prepare formula, how much to give, and how to establish a good feeding relationship.

WEANING GRADUALLY OR ABRUPTLY

Slow weaning, the generally preferred way of ending breastfeeding, is especially sensible with the older infant. Weaning gradually may be easier on your baby, especially if she is nursing a lot or seems to love nursing. Taking it slow may be easier on you, too. If your baby is going through a period of decreased interest in nursing, this may seem like a natural opportunity to stop nursing entirely. Still, you probably have established a large milk supply that can't be instantly shut down. Gradual weaning allows the breasts time to slow the production of milk painlessly, and also allows you time to observe your baby's reaction to formula. And because the immunological substances in breast milk increase in concentration with gradual weaning, you'll provide your baby increasing protection against infection as breastfeeding slowly comes to an end. Gradual weaning also allows you to change your mind. Sometimes mothers who begin weaning gradually discover that nursing less often is pleasurable, and so continue with less frequent breastfeeding for months or years.

A baby weaned from the breast before the end of her first year should be fed commercially prepared formula, not cow's milk. For reasons described in Chapter 2 (page 70), cow's milk—or goat's milk or homemade formula—is an inadequate food for a baby.

If your baby has never had formula or has had it only infrequently, it's important to determine that she can tolerate formula before you completely wean. If you gradually cut the number of daily nursings over a period of a few weeks, you'll have time to identify any problem and, if necessary, change your plans. If you want to wean more quickly, you can start out feeding formula exclusively, but you might express your milk for the first several days to maintain your milk supply in case your baby doesn't tolerate the formula. (Using a fully automatic electric breast pump can make expressing your milk easier and quicker. You can freeze the milk and offer it to your baby later.) Symptoms that a baby doesn't tolerate a certain formula may include bouts of crying, passing a lot of gas, increased spitting up or vomiting, rashes, redness around the rectum, and frequent watery stools that may be green, bloody, or contain mucus (soy formulas typically produce pale green, semi-formed stools). Some older babies who are weaned to formula get constipated. Wheezing and a stuffy or runny nose can indicate an allergy to formula.

If your baby does not seem to tolerate cow's-milk formula, check with your doctor about switching to a soy formula. Soy formula may not solve the problem, though, since one-third to one-half of all babies who are allergic to cow's-milk formulas are also allergic to soy (Bahna 1987). If your baby can't tolerate soy, the next option may be one of the "predigested," hypoallergenic formulas, which are very expensive.

More than a few mothers, having weaned to formulas only to find their babies couldn't tolerate any of them, have regretted giving up nursing. Some have even tried to relactate, which is not easy. This is why it is important to wean slowly, or to keep up your milk supply by using an electric pump, until you are sure you can give your baby formula without making her sick.

> As many as half of all babies who are allergic to cow's-milk formulas are also allergic to soy formulas.

Despite the often heard advice that weaning should proceed gradually, many mothers do wean all at once or over a period of just a few days. As a result they often suffer from breast pain caused by engorgement, which may last for several days. Most breasts take a while to get the message to stop producing milk, and in the meantime the milk within has nowhere to go. Abrupt weaning can cause "milk fever," with symptoms of engorgement, mild fever, aching, and fatigue lasting up to four days. Milk fever is thought to be caused by the re-absorption of milk into the body. (Antibiotics are unnecessary for treating milk fever, because the breast is not infected. Mastitis is distinguished by a reddened area of the breast as well as fever and other flu-like symptoms.)

If you are confident about your baby's ability to tolerate formula, and you are determined to stop milk production at once or you have no choice in the matter, you can either suffer through the engorgement, or you can nurse (or express milk) just enough to keep you comfortable. In either case your milk supply will drop. A supportive bra, mild pain relievers, and ice packs will help while you are engorged; so may chilled cabbage leaves in your bra and drinking sage tea (see page 67). If you need a stronger remedy, you might try vitamin B_6 or, in an emergency, the pre-scription drug Dostinex (see page 68). In the meantime, remove only as much milk as necessary. Unless you are weaning because you must take an unsafe medication, give any milk you collect to your baby. Your breasts will probably remain full and lumpy for five to ten days following complete weaning. This shouldn't be cause for concern unless your breast is red in any area and you experience fever and other flu-like symptoms. Occasionally a mother does develop a breast infection during weaning, in which case she is likely to require antibiotic therapy.

Mothers often ask about "dry-up" pills to end milk production. Until recently these medications were frequently prescribed after delivery for mothers who did not intend to breastfeed. As described in Chapter 2, however, the drugs can have potentially serious side effects, they can be quite expensive, and after the ten-day course of medication milk produc-tion frequently resumes (see page 68).

More gradual weaning has no hard and fast rules. In the weaning process are two main steps: substituting something else for each nurs-ing, and watching for any physical or emotional reaction in the baby or yourself. Generally, if your baby is mostly dependent on breast milk, you begin by replacing a day or evening nursing with formula. If you observe no reactions to the formula—such as rash, increased spitting up or vom-iting, bowel problems, crying bouts, wheezing, or nasal congestion—and if you don't feel engorged, after a few days or weeks you replace a second nursing. Ideally, you wean slowly enough to avoid an unhappy, clingy baby or full, uncomfortable breasts.

If at any time during the process you notice that the baby is not doing well on the formula, or you miss nursing and change your mind about weaning, several days of stepped-up nursing will probably rebuild your milk supply. See "Concerns about Your Milk Supply," page 36.

If your older baby is taking solid foods well, you can give up nursings before mealtimes, one meal at a time, and instead feed a cup of formula along with the meal. You can also slowly eliminate between-meal nursings, substituting a snack and formula.

The last nursings to go are usually the early-morning and sleep-time ones. These are easiest to eliminate by substituting a different activity for nursing. Although your baby may quickly give up the early-morning nursing if you get up early to make him breakfast, you may decide instead to continue nursing at this time so you can sleep a while longer. You may want to wait a while, too, before eliminating the bedtime and naptime nursings. These may be your favorite times of the day with your child, a time to wind down and cuddle together as he peacefully drifts off to sleep. Some mothers continue nursing at bedtime, naptime, or both for weeks or even months after omitting the other nursings, whereas others substitute a new sleep-time routine, like a bath, a massage, and a drink, to make the transition easier. Such a routine, along with cuddling, singing, or rocking, may help a baby fall asleep happily without the breast. In some families Dad takes over at bedtime to establish new routines that are not associated with nursing.

Even if you have eliminated nursings gradually, and have recently been nursing only once or twice a day, you may still experience engorgement for a week or so after the last feeding. You can best manage engorgement by wearing a supportive bra, taking mild pain relievers, drinking sage tea (see page 67), and applying ice packs or cabbage leaves to the breasts (see page 67). If you need more relief, nurse briefly, or express just a small amount of milk. You may experience a few days of "milk fever," too (see page 67). A reddened area of the breast, accompanied by fever and other flu-like symptoms, indicates a breast infection, which should be treated with antibiotics.

Regardless of whether you are weaning quickly or slowly, anticipate that your fertility will return soon, if it hasn't already. The decrease in nursing during the weaning process can stimulate ovulation. For most women, fertility returns within a month or two after final weaning.

SELECTING A FORMULA

Unless you have already offered your baby a certain formula that he seems to tolerate, you may be unsure of which one to try. There is no one "best" formula. Formulas for older babies come in four varieties: regular cow's milk–based, soybean-based, "follow-up," and "predigested" (see page 69). Your baby's doctor will probably recommend a regular cow's-milk formula unless there is reason to suspect that your baby has an allergy to cow's milk. If your baby reacted to dairy products in your diet during breastfeeding, or if someone else in your family has a milk allergy, try one of the soy formulas. As explained in Chapter 2, the brand of formula you choose probably doesn't matter much (see page 69).

Follow-up formula is designed for older babies who are eating a wide variety of soft foods. Based on cow's milk and fortified with iron, follow-up formula is approximately 20 percent less expensive than regular infant formulas. Although advertisements might lead parents to think that follow-up formula is somehow better for older babies, it does not offer nutritional advantages over regular formulas. Follow-up formula contains the same number of calories as regular formula, but the fat content is less. For this reason a baby should be well established on a wide variety of other foods before follow-up formula is considered.

"Predigested" formulas are intended for those infants who are intolerant of both cow's-milk and soy formulas. "Predigested" formulas are very expensive.

Formula made from cow's milk is available in both low-iron and iron-fortified forms. Soy formulas are all iron-fortified. As explained in Chapter 2 (page 69), feeding babies iron-fortified formula prevents iron deficiency. A baby who isn't breastfeeding needs iron-fortified formula even if he is eating an iron-fortified cereal, since iron from cereal may not be absorbed well.

For information on the various kinds of formula, mixing formula, and the cost of formula, see "Selecting a Formula" in Chapter 2 (page 69).

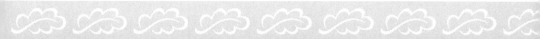

WEANING TO A BOTTLE OR CUP

Although most mothers who stop nursing before their babies reach twelve months wean to a bottle, this is not the only choice or necessarily the best one. Unless well controlled by parents, the bottle can become a child's constant companion and, as we'll see, a threat to her health. Besides, a baby weaned to a bottle must usually be weaned from it later on. Still, weaning to a bottle is sometimes necessary. Babies can handle a cup at about six months of age, but many are unable at that age to consume from the cup alone as much milk as they require, and therefore they need a bottle. By eight to ten months, most babies are able to take sufficient amounts of milk from a cup. If you can wait that long, you probably won't need a bottle.

If your baby has had bottles recently she should have little trouble accepting one. Advice on bottle feeding a baby who has never had bottles, or who objects to the whole idea, can be found in Chapter 2 (page 73). Information on bottle and nipple selection can also be found in Chapter 2 (page 72).

It helps to use breastfeeding as the model for bottle feeding. The tendency of breastfed babies to develop higher intellectual ability may stem partly from the frequent and prolonged contact they have with their mothers (see page 21). Babies who hold their own bottles lose some very important contact and stimulation. Sometimes a bottle and rubber nipple become a baby's main comfort in life.

Besides tempting parents away from the nurturing interaction their baby needs during feedings, the bottle can become unhealthful in other ways. Babies often drop bottles and then put them back in their mouths; this is a common cause of formula contamination and, probably, resulting sickness. Older babies and toddlers who get used to carrying bottles around with them or are put to sleep with the bottle are at risk for developing nursing caries, which can require major dental work. Ear infections can result when babies lie flat on their backs to suck from bottles. Dependence on a bottle can also lead to overconsumption of formula or juice, and lack of interest in other foods.

If you wean to a bottle, then, stay in control of it. Make a commitment to hold your baby in your arms whenever you feed her, and have your mate and other caregivers do the same. Doing so will be well worth your time.

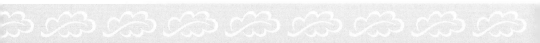

If your baby persistently refuses to make friends with an artificial nipple, or if you would prefer to forego the bottle, you might consider weaning to a cup instead. You can safely skip the bottle if your baby is able to drink a few ounces at a time from a cup. If she is able to take only an ounce or two at a time, you might consider slowing the pace of weaning until she is able to drink more from a cup. In a month or so, with daily practice at mealtimes, she will get the hang of drinking from a cup and will be able to take more.

Many parents offer their babies fluids from "training cups," which have tight-fitting lids and spouts. Although training cups may be easier for some babies to manage and are certainly less messy for parents, occasionally substituting a regular cup will help a baby learn to drink rather than suck.

At first, your baby will probably be unable to manage a cup by herself. Once she does begin holding her own cup, be prepared for her turning it over to see what happens. This is all part of the learning process.

PREPARING FORMULA

Formula, unlike breast milk, offers an infant no protective antibodies. The formula-fed baby is therefore more susceptible to pathogens—and he is also more likely to be exposed to them. Germs can easily be transmitted from the hands of the feeder, rubber nipples, bottles, formula, water, and any utensils used in preparing and feeding formula. Any of these things may be contaminated if great care isn't taken in formula preparation and feeding.

Many health-care providers have developed a casual attitude about formula preparation. But formula-fed infants commonly get sick and sometimes must be hospitalized because of gastrointestinal infections. This may be partially because babies get no immunological protection from formula, but also partially because bottles and formula are carelessly prepared and handled.

Because an older baby's immune system is more mature than a young baby's, sterilizing bottles and formula is probably unnecessary. Nevertheless, when preparing bottles it is important that all of the feeding equipment, including your sink and bottle brush, be very clean. Keep these rules in mind:

◆ Use a dishwasher only if the water reaches a temperature of about 140 degrees F. Wash the bottles using the full cycle, including pre-rinse.

◆ Boil the nipples, and keep them in a clean, dry, covered container.

◆ Always wash off the top of the formula can with hot, soapy water, and rinse it well before opening it with a clean, punch-type can opener.

◆ When preparing formula using nonsterile techniques, prepare each bottle just before each feeding.

◆ Make sure you have pure water for mixing formula. Read "Evaluating Your Water Supply" in Chapter 2 (pages 78-80).

A warning about mixing formula: A study found that half of home-mixed formula bottles are mixed incorrectly, with either too much formula or too much water (McJunkin et al. 1987). As explained in Chapter 2, it is very important to follow the directions carefully when mixing liquid concentrate or powdered formula. Careless mixing can make a baby sick.

Read and follow the directions on measuring the powder. Do not shake or tap the side of the measuring scoop; level the powder by using the flat edge of a knife. When measuring water or liquid concentrate, use a clear glass measuring cup, and measure accurately.

For information on safely storing formula and warming bottles, see Chapter 2, pages 80-81.

HOW MUCH TO FEED

Four- to Eight-Month-Olds

The amounts of formula and solid foods your baby takes are best determined by your baby. They will depend on his age and growth pattern, his activity level, and other factors such as illness. By and large, babies can be trusted to take as much as they need as often as they need it. This section, however, provides general feeding guidelines based on the needs of the average baby.

Most four- to six-month-olds take about 32 ounces of breast milk or formula per day; some take less. To estimate the formula needs of a baby who is not taking solids, multiply the baby's weight in pounds by 2.5. The result expresses the number of ounces of formula a four- to six-month-old baby needs each day, to a maximum of 32 ounces of formula.

Babies usually start eating solids between ages four and seven months, when they become developmentally ready for them and begin to benefit from them nutritionally. Iron-fortified infant cereal mixed with breast milk or formula is a good first food for a baby, since it is easy to swallow and digest and may help meet the baby's increased need for iron that occurs around six months. Mixing the cereal with breast milk or formula provides a good combination of carbohydrates, protein, and fat. You can adjust the texture of the cereal by using varying amounts of milk to match your baby's ability with semi-soft foods. You might offer cereal once or twice a day, increasing the amount from just a teaspoon or so at first to a half-cup per day. During this period, offer solids only after feedings of breast milk or formula.

Milk or formula remains a baby's most important food until she is eating three regular meals a day, some time after eight months of age.

After your baby is taking about a half-cup of cereal a day, you can add fruits and vegetables to her diet. Although commercially prepared fruits and vegetables are nutritionally adequate, pureed types do not accustom a baby to different textures or help her learn chewing skills. Jars of baby food are also a waste of money. Fresh or frozen fruits, or canned fruits

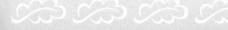

packed in water, and fresh or frozen vegetables, or vegetables canned without salt, are more economical. They can be mashed, scraped, diced, or chunked according to a baby's ability. An inexpensive baby-food grinder may be a worthwhile purchase. A meal pattern that may work well during this period is cereal and fruit in the morning, and cereal and vegetable in the evening. You might start with one to two tablespoons of fruit or vegetable per day, and gradually increase the amount to one-third cup a day.

As your baby increases her intake of cereal, fruits, and vegetables, her milk needs will generally drop. Regardless of whether you decide to wean to a bottle, it is a good idea to offer a cup to your baby at mealtimes beginning when she is about six months old. Many older babies take much or all of their formula from a cup. If you offer a cup at mealtimes, your baby will be able to wean from the bottle at around twelve months.

Juices should be limited to 3 ounces a day. "Juice abuse" is a common mistake in infant feeding. Overdependence on juice can cause a baby to take too little milk or solid foods, suffer with diarrhea, and, especially if the juice is given in a bottle, end up with decayed teeth. Juices are probably best offered from a cup. Avoid "fruit drinks," which are water and corn syrup or sugar with some juice added. Acidic juices, such as orange, pineapple, and tomato, can lead to allergic reactions in many babies.

During the period from four to eight months you can also offer your baby breads, crackers, dry cereals, pasta, rice, and other cooked grains. These provide B vitamins and iron as well as calories. Although she may not actually eat much at first, your baby will be developing her chewing and self-feeding skills.

Try not to worry if your baby eats very little before she is eight months old. She will have her own food preferences, and they will change often. She may refuse a certain food one week and happily eat it the next. She may refuse all foods for a while if she is not feeling well. And, as she asserts her independence, she may also turn her head at any food offered from a spoon. Despite the inevitable mess, you should let her feed herself. Give her a spoon or allow her to use her fingers. Let her examine her food, if she wants, before she decides whether to eat it. By feeding herself, your baby will develop her grasping skills and hand-eye coordination. Be patient if she plays with her food instead of eating it; keep in mind that during this period breast milk or formula (depending on where you are in the weaning process) continues to be the most important part of her diet.

Eight- to Twelve-Month-Olds

Between eight and ten months of age, if not before, your baby will probably become interested in what the rest of the family is eating. Once table foods are offered, three major transitions follow:

◆ The first transition is adding another meal or two so the baby is eating three to four meals a day.

◆ The second transition is adding high-protein foods as the baby's intake of milk drops.

◆ The last transition is providing the meal before breastfeeding, or giving formula along with the meal or afterward, depending on where you are in the weaning process. This encourages the baby to take more solids.

Most eight- to ten-month-olds take about 26 to 30 ounces of milk or formula per day. Most ten- to twelve-month-olds take a little less—about 22 to 28 ounces of milk or formula per day.

This new meal pattern basically requires the addition of a midday meal and, perhaps, a small snack. Continuing to give a half-cup of cereal over the course of one or two meals (or one meal and a snack) is still a good idea. Two other servings of grains (which can include bread, crackers, dry cereals, pasta, rice, and other cooked grains) complete the baby's requirements for these. You should probably offer a fruit or vegetable at each meal, about one to two tablespoons per serving. Juice may substitute for one serving, but should still be limited to about 3 ounces a day.

The baby older than eight months should also be offered at least two servings of high-protein foods every day (a serving of meat, poultry, fish, or eggs is about one tablespoon, or one-half ounce). Although chicken and fish, carefully boned, are fairly easy for a baby to manage, red meats

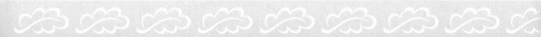

must usually be shredded, ground, or minced. Avoid lunch meats and hot dogs, which are high in salt and nitrates. If allergies are a concern, cook eggs until solid, and offer only the yolks. Other high-protein foods for a baby of this age include hard cheese and cottage cheese, tofu, shell beans, peas, and lentils. Commercially prepared "infant dinners" are a poor source of protein, being mostly vegetables and water with a small amount of meat.

If you prefer that your child has a vegetarian diet, this is easy so long as you include cheese and eggs. Do take the time to learn all you can about vegetarian nutrition and the nutritional needs of infants and toddlers; two books that can get you started are *Child of Mine* and *The New Laurel's Kitchen* (see References). You might also want to consult with a nutritionist, especially if you are considering a vegan (vegetable-only) diet. Young children on such diets are at substantial risk for B-vitamin deficiencies and, because of a lack of protein, general growth deficiencies. The federal Special Supplemental Nutrition Program for Women, Infants, and Children (WIC) or your local public health department can probably refer you to a nutritionist for further guidance.

Although your baby probably won't eat precisely the suggested amounts of grains, fruits, vegetables, and high-protein foods every day, weekly averages close to the recommended amounts will ensure he is well nourished. If by eight to ten months your baby continues to take solids only sporadically at best, it may be time to give him a little extra encouragement. If his growth falls off, and, perhaps, he seems to be sick a lot, he may be getting overly dependent on the breast or bottle, and substituting nursing or bottle feeding for eating a variety of nutritious foods. In this case, make sure you are nursing or bottle feeding after meals, not before. Always include the baby in family meals, but offer food at other times if he refuses it at mealtimes. If he resents your pushing solids, have someone else feed him or let him feed himself.

Never assume because he spits something out one day that your baby won't take it the next.

If you've completed the process just described, you have made good progress in weaning by expanding your baby's diet to include other foods. Perhaps you've already weaned completely, or perhaps you'll continue to find nursing convenient for early-morning feedings, snacks, naps, bedtime, and general soothing and comforting. Sooner or later, slowly or quickly, you and your child will eliminate some or all of these nursings by substituting other foods, beverages, or activities.

four

WEANING YOUR ONE- OR TWO-YEAR-OLD

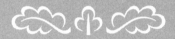

AFTER A YEAR OR MORE OF BREASTFEEDING, you probably feel proud of all you've given your baby, and rightly so. But now she isn't such a baby anymore. You may have specific reasons to consider ending breastfeeding, or you may simply feel that this is the right time to wean.

IS IT TIME TO WEAN?

Continued nursing has considerable benefits for a toddler. Breast milk retains nutritional and immunological values throughout the course of lactation. As a mother's milk output declines with gradual weaning, in fact, some nutrients—including protein and fat—and immunological components become more concentrated in the milk (Dewey 1984, Garza et al. 1983, Goldman 1983, Mandel et al. 2005). This may help ensure the health of children whose diets are restricted by a lack of suitable adult foods.

Nursing also helps a toddler get to sleep easily (which prompts some mothers to call their milk "knock-out drops") and to wake up gently. Nursing helps the toddler deal with hurts, both physical and emotional, and provides solace after encounters with strangers, crowds, and all the new and frightening experiences of the toddler's daily life. Because nursing helps a toddler to maintain an intimate connection with the person she needs most, many employed mothers feel it is especially important to continue nursing their children beyond the first year. Finally, in the opinion of many mothers, nursing beyond infancy makes for a confident, sociable child who cares more about people than things.

Does nursing beyond infancy pose any harm to the child? Many people think that a nursing toddler is too emotionally dependent on her mother. If you have a shy or clingy child, rest assured that nursing hasn't made her that way. Allowing your child the security of blissful interludes at your breasts, in fact, can only strengthen her for dealings with the big, cruel world. If you're patient now, she'll probably grow out of her shyness. In a year or two, people she meets may never guess she was once timid.

Doctors used to say that nursing beyond infancy makes a child weak and sickly. You may wonder if this is true, particularly if your child takes little food besides your milk. Actually, nursing children between the ages of sixteen and thirty months have been found to have fewer and briefer illnesses than other children their age (Gulick 1986). The World Health Organization maintains that "a modest increase in breastfeeding rates could prevent up to 10 percent of all deaths of children under five." If a rare child becomes too dependent on breast milk, this problem is likely to vanish when a variety of nutritious and easily digested foods are offered several times a day. Even most nursing toddlers who refuse all solids are plump, healthy children. They may be responding naturally to late dental development or allergies.

Even if you know nursing is good for your toddler, you may have the nagging feeling that you're missing some deadline. "It's now or never!" your friends may say, when you tell them you're thinking about weaning your one-year-old. Some people talk about "windows for weaning," when a child's interest in the breast naturally wanes. One of these windows, according to T. Berry Brazelton (1983), is between ages nine and twelve months. Other people give you until eighteen months; beyond that, they say, weaning gets much harder. If your child is one and a half or two, you may wonder if you've made a big mistake. Will your child *ever* wean?

Although it's true that many children are easily distracted from nursing from the time they can crawl or "cruise"—walking along while hanging onto furniture or people—most very much need to return now and then to the security, the bliss, of sucking at the breast. The more daring their explorations, in fact, the more reassuring contact they need.

A child's second and third years are a challenging, frustrating time for her, as she struggles to walk, talk, reach, climb, control her urine and bowel movements, work alongside her elders, and simply *get her own way*, to be defeated again by her own ineptness or fears, or by the bigger people around her. She may feel competitive with older, abler siblings, who are granted privileges she is forbidden. And if another baby comes along, her whole basis of security is undermined.

Between about nine and eighteen months, a child is in a phase of not only intrepid exploration but also intense separation anxiety. As she struggles to achieve mobility and elemental communication skills, she becomes more and more acutely aware of how much she depends on her parents. Nursing becomes increasingly important to her during these months; she seems to feel that it restores her attachment to her mother. In a study of children in various societies, an anthropologist found adverse reactions to weaning strongest in children between thirteen and eighteen months old. Beyond eighteen months, reactions grew milder with age (Waletsky 1977). Children vary in their rates of development, of course, but if your child panics every time you leave a room without her she is definitely not ready to wean.

You may wonder if it's time to wean because your child is beginning to walk or talk. You've probably heard people say that a child is too old for the breast if she can ask for it. In many societies, developmental milestones, such as eruption of teeth, walking, and talking, are considered signals to wean. It's certainly more sensible to time weaning by a child's individual development than by her chronological age. Parents have to be careful, though, in deciding when a milestone has been reached. Children develop in alternating phases of inwardness and expansiveness. Periods of confidence and easy mastery of skills alternate with periods of struggle, apparent stagnancy, and even backsliding. A child who has just taken her first steps may still be a long way from her next developmental plateau; she'll take plenty of falls before she can walk with ease and grace. When she can walk easily, though, you might say she has truly reached a milestone. She is likely to be calmer and happier for a while, and to make sudden strides in her verbal and social development as well.

One developmental step parents find particularly helpful in weaning occurs when toddlers begin to sleep more deeply. Although we've found no scientific studies on this subject, the change seems to occur around the age of two and a half. Suddenly, you may find, you can transfer your sleeping child from the car, backpack, or stroller to the bed, and she doesn't wake up (provided you're gentle and the house is quiet). It becomes much easier at this point to get a child to bed without nursing, and she may also sleep for longer stretches.

If you're looking for a "window for weaning," then, consider your child's stage of development, how she is behaving, and how she seems to feel. Make sure she is not only emotionally at ease but also physically healthy, since sickness and even teething can make weaning very difficult. Consider outside influences, too, such as the availability of loved ones who can distract her from the breast by providing attention and affection, and even the weather—trying to wean while you're stuck indoors for the winter may not be worth the trouble. Remember that, in general, the older your child gets the easier weaning will be. Keep this in mind, too: If your child becomes overanxious or depressed during weaning, you can always give up weaning for a while, and try again a few months later.

WILL YOUR TODDLER SELF-WEAN?

Many women put off weaning their toddlers in the hope that they will soon stop nursing on their own. Although it has often been said that most children will self-wean between ages two and four, this isn't borne out by the experiences of women we know. A few toddlers do decide to stop nursing; one thirteen-month-old, already down to one or two nursings per day, spit out the nipple one day, said, "Blehhhh," and never nursed again. Another child, the same age, laughed at her mother's bare breast, and likewise never nursed again. But such behavior is unusual, according to Ruth Lawrence, author of a leading breastfeeding guide for physicians. Children rarely initiate weaning between the ages of one and four years, Lawrence says (1989, 253). The mother who claims her toddler self-weaned is usually forgetting the encouragement she gave—for example, by offering food and drink instead of the breast, by distracting the child with books and play, and by postponing nursings. Without strong encouragement, children are highly unlikely to stop nursing before they are through the toddler years.

This doesn't mean weaning a toddler must be difficult or traumatic for you both. It just means that the axiom "Don't offer, don't refuse" probably won't bring an end to nursing for many months to come. If you want to stop nursing before your child reaches age three or four, you will probably need to make a conscious decision to do so. And if your child nurses avidly or has a demanding temperament, you will probably have to work hard at bringing an end to breastfeeding. You may decide instead to keep nursing until your child is about three, when weaning will probably become much easier (see Chapter 5). In the meantime, you may be able to reduce nursings to a more tolerable frequency, perhaps just twice a day, at naptime and bedtime.

ARE *YOU* READY TO WEAN?

Nursing past infancy, or giving up nursing, affects not only a child's well-being but also his mother's. Before deciding to bring about an end to nursing, you'll want to consider the pros and the cons of weaning for you, and sort out your feelings on the matter.

If you have been nursing without restriction (and without both the use of bottles or pacifiers and lengthy separations from your child), you may still be enjoying freedom from the menstrual cycle—from the fluctuations in mood, appetite, weight, and so on; from the pain of menstrual cramps; from the cost of buying tampons or sanitary pads; from the bother of using them. How long, you may wonder, can this freedom continue? A mother who nurses without restriction, during the night as well as the day, can usually expect a period of lactational amenorrhea lasting one to two years (Stern et al. 1986). This period tends to be longer, one study found, in women who are younger, who are slender, who gained plenty of weight in pregnancy, who produce more milk, and who have more children (Heinig et al. 1994). After a nursing mother resumes her periods, menstrual symptoms may still be moderated by lactation hormones.

Ovulation usually occurs shortly before, or within a few months after, menstruation resumes. If you are still amenorrheic in the second year of nursing, you will probably ovulate, and thereby become fertile, *before* you have your first period. A small minority of women, however, never ovulate while they are nursing. If you want your children's births closely spaced, you may decide to wean so you can get pregnant again.

Other benefits of nursing past infancy are the decreased risks of developing cancer of the breast and other organs (Fackelmann 1992), the tranquilizing effect of the hormone oxytocin (produced in response to the baby's sucking), the opportunities to rest, read, or even nap during the day, and the ease in comforting a sick, teething, or upset child and in getting the child to sleep. Some toddlers refuse to take naps if they can't nurse to sleep, and are cranky every afternoon as a result.

The enlarged breasts of a nursing mother may be an advantage or disadvantage, depending on your preference. After weaning, your breasts will probably be smaller than they were before you got pregnant.

If you are still over your prepregnant weight, you may or may not lose the extra pounds upon ending breastfeeding. Some women report losing several pounds within a week following their last nursing. Your appetite and energy needs will certainly decline during and after weaning. If you eat according to habit rather than appetite, you may actually gain weight during this time, as many women do.

If you have been prone to breast infections, they may continue in the second and third years even if you nurse only a few times each day. Weaning will of course put an end to these bouts, although you *can* get mastitis in the first few days after the last nursing, especially if you wean abruptly.

A possible disadvantage of nursing after a baby's first year is having to face the disapproval of others. Against the recommendations of the American Academy of Pediatrics, the American Dietetic Association, and the World Health Organization, almost two-thirds of U.S. babies are completely weaned by the age of six months. Many women who breastfeed longer do so only in secret, and so promote the general view of breastfeeding past the first year as deviant. Openly nursing a toddler may seem no big deal, depending on where you live and who your friends are. In 2004, for example, over a quarter of U.S. college graduates nursed their babies for at least a year, as did 35 percent of mothers in the Seattle area. But in some circles people may see nursing a walking, talking child as unconventional, unnecessary, and embarrassing. They probably won't openly challenge or criticize you, but you may feel their silent disapproval. If you want to continue nursing, you may find strength in reading this book and others on breastfeeding, talking with breastfeeding advocates, such as La Leche League members, and looking into your own heart. Develop friendships with women who raise their children in the way you'd like to raise yours. Talk openly about breastfeeding if it helps to clear the air, or keep it secret if you really must (see "Nursing in Public," page 129).

There are without doubt some clear advantages to weaning. "I'm so glad to have my body back," many women say, meaning their bodies no longer seem to belong to their babies. One mother remarked on how nice it was to cuddle with her child without feeling she was "under assault." After weaning you can again wear shirts that tuck in, without continually having to untuck them, and dresses without frontal openings. You may be able to get away from home by yourself for a few hours, or even a few days, without your child totally falling apart. After a period of adjustment following weaning, your toddler will probably sleep in longer stretches and more willingly accept comfort from Daddy or someone else. If your toddler isn't drinking at night, you'll have an easier time getting her to stay dry in bed. And after weaning you may find more opportunity, and inclination, for intimacy with your mate.

All the benefits of weaning will come in time, of course, and you may decide that you can wait for them. But, if you are like most women, the decision whether to wean may be complicated by your own ambivalence. You're probably attracted to the real and the imagined benefits of weaning; you may envision yourself as active, slim, well rested, and well dressed, with free arms and a back that never aches. But perhaps you also can't let go of that other vision, of yourself in a tender embrace with a warm, sweet-smelling baby. This is no soft-focus marketing image; you know the joy of watching your child suck away into deep slumber, or feeling her snuggle against you in bed on a cold morning. You know that nursing makes life easier for you; at any moment, you can give your child instant consolation and a quiet escape into sleep. You may fear hurting your child by denying what she naturally desires, and feel guilty about wanting more freedom. Your toddler has similar feelings: She wants independence from you one minute and craves your comforting breast the next. All change, of course, entails some loss. And change is inevitable; your child *will* grow up and stop nursing. How and when weaning happens is for you to determine. There is no one right time and way to wean. Acknowledging this, and accepting your mixed feelings, will help you keep your actions firm and clear. Consistency in your behavior will give your child confidence, and so make whatever path you take smoother for both of you.

This doesn't mean you must now plan and schedule a complete course of weaning. In the following section we discuss problems that are frequently considered reasons for weaning a toddler. Many women who consult Kathleen for help with weaning continue nursing after such problems are resolved. For you, resolving one or more of these problems may entail complete weaning, or may instead allow you to nurse happily for many months to come.

Possible Reasons to Wean Your Toddler

PREGNANT AGAIN

If you're having sex and not using any form of birth control, you're likely to become pregnant when nursing sessions have declined to fewer than about six a day, or less than eighty minutes total, during your child's first eighteen months. After eighteen months to two years, your periods, and your fertility, may return despite frequent suckling (Stern et al. 1986).

Many women believe pregnancy necessitates weaning, though they may have no clear idea why it should. They may have a vague notion that the milk would be bad for the child, or that there would be no milk, or that the fetus would be deprived. These ideas date to Aristotle, whose assertion that women don't conceive while nursing, and that if they do the milk dries up, was referred to by writers on infant care and nutrition for over two millennia afterward, and also to the age-old popular belief that breast milk is formed from menstrual blood not shed in pregnancy (Fildes 1986, 20).

If you have experienced preterm labor, your doctor will probably advise against nursing (or having sex) during pregnancy. Otherwise, continuing to breastfeed shouldn't hurt your fetus or your nursing toddler, and if your diet is very good it won't hurt you, either. But you may find it quite uncomfortable. In a study of La Leche League members who became pregnant while nursing, 74 percent of the mothers reported pain in the nipples or breast (Newton and Theotokas 1979). For some women the pain is minor; they can easily bear it by breathing deeply to help themselves relax, or by distracting themselves, perhaps with a book. Others find the pain harder to bear, and must fight to stifle their gasps or moans through each nursing.

Pregnancy may affect nursing in other ways, too. In the Newton and Theotokas study, nearly 20 percent of the women felt a general restlessness while nursing, and 17 percent felt irritation at the nursing child. Sixty-five percent noticed, during the first four months of pregnancy, a decrease in the milk supply. Women who feel a stronger sex drive during pregnancy may be disturbed by feelings of arousal while nursing. And in late pregnancy breastfeeding may increase the strength and frequency of Braxton-Hicks contractions—although nursing *won't* cause premature labor.

Symptoms such as restlessness, irritability, reduced milk supply, and sexual arousal are caused by hormonal changes in pregnancy (some women notice similar symptoms about the time their periods start). Because these symptoms can make nursing during pregnancy so unpleasant, you might think of them as nature's way of telling you to stop— or, as Newton and Theotokas put it, as "a psychobiological weaning mechanism." In fact, although the women Newton and Theotokas studied presumably subscribed to La Leche's philosophy of child-led weaning, 69 percent of them weaned during pregnancy.

Some of their children may have weaned themselves. Many toddlers choose to wean during their mothers' pregnancies, either because of the decrease in the milk supply or because of the change in the taste of the milk, when, during late pregnancy, it becomes colostrum. Other children continue nursing avidly despite these changes:

> *I asked her several times, "Is there any milk left?" "Oh yes, Mommy, there's lots of milk!" Everything was fine with her. She was able to talk about it. So finally at the end of the pregnancy, "Cornelia," I said, "You've really been telling Mommy a lot of jokes, haven't you? There's really not any milk left." She said, "No there really isn't. But I still need to sit close to you" (Owen 1989, 93–94).*

Some toddlers nurse even more during pregnancy than they did before, possibly to get enough milk to satisfy them, or from insecurity because a new rival is on the way, or from anxiety caused by the mother's restlessness and crying with the pain of sore nipples.

Some breastfeeding counselors recommend coping with the pain of nursing in pregnancy through Lamaze breathing, relaxation techniques, or airing the nipples. But these measures are unlikely to make nursing really comfortable. Many mothers want to continue nursing for the child's sake, especially if the pregnancy was unplanned and, in the mother's opinion, premature. Some women manage by limiting the frequency of nursings, or the length of each nursing. If a woman can't stay quiet and calm as she nurses, though, complete weaning may be wiser. A child feels great sadness when she knows she is hurting her mother. It makes no sense for a mother to prolong the pain—hers *and* her child's—out of guilt feelings.

Some mothers just explain the problem to their toddlers. "I have bad owies on my chi chis, I can't nurse you anymore," said one. "I'm going to hold you and snuggle with you but it hurts too much to nurse" (Owen 1989, 80). Most toddlers can understand this, and will try hard to comply. They need a lot of extra cuddling at this time, though, as well as distractions like books and walks, and substitutions like snacks in the night.

Giving up nursing a child during pregnancy doesn't necessarily mean cutting that child off from the breast forever. Sometimes a toddler who stops nursing during pregnancy starts again after the baby is born, when, as one little girl said, "There's enough milk for everybody!" (Owen 1989, 94). A toddler may resume nursing, if allowed, even after months without the breast.

Some women wean not because they are pregnant but because they want to get pregnant. A small proportion of mothers must wean completely for their menstrual cycles to resume.

Sometimes a nursing woman experiences little discomfort in pregnancy, and may actually enjoy nursing during these months. Nursing gives her opportunities to lie down and relax, and lets her prolong the closeness she has had with her toddler, who may otherwise have been prematurely banished from babyhood. If pregnancy happens to end in miscarriage, nursing helps the mother work through her grief. And if the baby is born too premature to suck, the nursing toddler might assist in keeping up the milk supply.

The thought of nursing two children at once makes many women shudder. "Tandem nursing," however, may not be as overwhelming as it sounds. Seventy-seven percent of the mothers in Newton and Theotokas's study who nursed two at once said they would "definitely" or "probably" do it again if they became pregnant while nursing. Such women say tandem nursing alleviates rivalry and helps build a strong bond between siblings. Other mothers complain that their toddlers want to nurse more after the new baby comes, and that they themselves feel resentment against the older nursing child. If you find you don't like tandem nursing, of course, you can always work at weaning your toddler *after* the baby comes.

NURSING IN PUBLIC

Many women want to wean their babies as soon as they start walking (or start talking, or turn one year old), if not before, because they are afraid of other people's looks, remarks, and general disapproval. For many women, this is a reason not to breastfeed at all; in a survey of Toronto mothers, most who chose to bottle-feed were uncomfortable with the idea of being seen breastfeeding, even by close friends in the mother's own home (Maclean 1990, 29). When a woman is comfortable nursing in public, her mate may still discourage it, because of his own feelings of embarrassment or jealousy.

By now, of course, you know how to nurse discreetly. Still, people in your community may be uncomfortable even knowing that you are nursing a toddler. This may or may not make *you* uncomfortable. If it does, nursing may be something you're willing to do only at home, with no one but close family members present.

With many toddlers, keeping nursing private is no problem. Since most toddlers nurse more for comfort than hunger, they are often able to wait a while for the breast, especially if they are over two years old. And many prefer to nurse in private. Some toddlers are happy nursing nowhere but on Mama's bed, or on the family couch, or wherever the favorite nursing spot is. Instead of tearing at your shirt in public, your toddler may pull on your hand and say, "Home!" If you are staying with friends or relatives, a private bedroom will probably be the next best place to nurse, from your child's point of view. Retire there, explaining that you need to put the baby to sleep (which you may well do). If she reappears with you a half hour later, just say she wasn't sleepy after all.

Some toddlers aren't so easy to satisfy, however. Your child may demand to nurse often no matter where you are or what you are doing. You may be able to negotiate with her, though, especially if she is over two. Some mothers tell their toddlers they won't be nursing at Grandma's, or in stores, or, perhaps, anywhere but at home. Some toddlers can accept this. If you make such a rule, however, you will have to make sure that you're in an allowed place at favorite nursing times, and that you are prepared with substitutes or distractions for other times. Adjusting to such limits may be hard for your child, but probably preferable to giving up nursing altogether. Repeating the rule firmly and applying it consistently will help your child adjust.

"Use your words," some parents tell their young children. You may regret this command if the word your child uses—loudly and publicly—is *boobies* or the like. Invent a code word for nursing, or encourage your child to use one that she has invented herself.

You may dislike public nursing because your child insists on exposing your whole chest. If she seems to feel smothered by your bulky sweater, you should probably take it off, but you can insist on keeping your shirt modestly down even at home. Make it clear your clothes are not for her to strip off whenever she feels like it.

Maybe you don't mind nursing in public now and then, but are bothered because your toddler puts her hand down your shirt whenever strangers are around. It may help to keep handy something else your toddler can hold to feel secure—something that requires two hands, like a large apple or a spill-proof cup. Complete weaning probably *won't* help with this problem—the breast-holding habit may continue for many months after suckling stops.

Some mothers nurse whenever and wherever their toddlers need it, and ignore what other people think. Although many people disapprove of nursing children over a year old, most haven't the nerve to say so. One woman noticed her parents' friends sometimes got up and left the room when she nursed, but she didn't let it bother her (Owen 1989, 47). Linda once nursed a two-year-old while testifying in court, and no one present made any comment. Most people who are uncomfortable in the presence of a nursing woman are embarrassed, not disgusted. You may come to see yourself as a pioneer, opening up new cultural territory. By boldly nursing in public you can help people overcome their awkward feelings, and make life easier for the women and children who follow you.

THE NONSTOP NURSER

Your toddler may be the sort who wants to nurse every half-hour or more, no matter where you are or what you're doing, and no matter how well he eats at the table. This doesn't bother some women; the !Kung people of the Kalahari Desert nurse about five times an hour during a child's first two years. But it may drive *you* crazy.

Nonstop nursers often have busy moms with older children. Such a toddler may demand the breast as a way of getting your attention. He may want to nurse whenever you sit down to talk on the phone, pay bills, use the computer, or play a board game with the older kids. If the child was an "easy" baby who seldom hampered your work much, this behavior may come as an unpleasant surprise. But if you often give in and nurse instead of finding other ways to keep him happy, you may be encouraging the bothersome behavior. Even if you consciously taught your child to nurse at such times, by offering the breast to keep him quiet, you may want to break the habit now. Perhaps one-handed typing with a tiny baby at your breast was no trouble, but with a squirming, kicking twenty-five-pounder on your lap it is surely harder.

Maybe you're nursing more than you want because of pressure from others. A woman from a large household complained that when she tried to wean her daughter, "Everybody would get so down on me. 'That baby's screaming, shut her up!'"(Owen 1989, 45). Your mate may tell you your toddler is "hungry" when he doesn't want to take the time to comfort the child; your older children may demand that you nurse the toddler so he will leave them and their Legos alone.

When your toddler is pounding your chest or tearing at your shirt, you can't appease him without nursing. But you may have been able to prevent this behavior by anticipating his needs. Or, once you start nursing, you may be able to cut the session short. Sometimes when you take your toddler off to nurse, he may stop after a few sucks to say, "Read book!" or to pull a blanket over his head, initiating a game of peek-a-boo. You probably get annoyed, especially if you thought he was going to take a nap. It helps to realize that what he may need at this moment is not to nurse *or* sleep, but to play and talk with you. After a short play or reading session he may happily go to sleep, or even play by himself for a while.

Evenings with your toddler may be hardest. The few hours between dinner and bed are busy times in today's households. Besides weekends, evenings are the only opportunities many couples have to talk, do chores, and take care of household business. If older children are away during the day, this time may also be their chance to talk with their parents and get help with their studies. And where does the toddler fit in? Chances are he gets lost in the shuffle.

When your toddler wants to nurse in the evening, you may feel initial relief. Finally, you think, he's going to go to sleep! After half an hour of playing and sucking he's almost out—but then the older kids come tearing in, yelling. You yell back and send them out, persuade the now wide-awake toddler to lie down, and start nursing again. Ten minutes later your mate marches in to summon you to the phone. You say you'll call back. But now the toddler is trying to do a headstand on the bed. Your five-year-old comes in to ask you to read to her. The toddler climbs off the bed and runs to get a book of his own. You fall asleep, but only momentarily. The toddler is back, really tired now and crying. You read a page or two, then nurse him briefly, and he starts to fall asleep. But then your mate throws open the door on his way to the bathroom, urinates noisily, and finishes with a roaring flush. The toddler sits up and looks around, but thankfully goes back to business. You're almost asleep when he releases the nipple. Then your five-year-old comes in crying. . . .

If your toddler is nursing for attention, weaning completely probably won't solve your problems. Whereas now you can usually satisfy him with the breast while you talk or read a novel, when he is weaned you'll have a more active parenting role—reading books to *him*, helping him assemble puzzles, putting together the train set. And if you don't give him enough attention, he may retreat inward by taking up thumb-sucking, or transfer his dependence to objects like a bottle, a pacifier, or even the television.

So how do you keep your toddler and the rest of your family happy without losing your mind? Getting through these years is much easier with some planning, a sense of fun, and plenty of help from your mate or friends. At least once a day, if possible, get someone else to keep your other kids company while you give your toddler your full attention.

Reserve any time that the toddler is asleep, and you're not, for writing, paying bills, using the computer, and so on. At times when you have to concentrate on such things while your toddler is awake, bring out a special basket of toys that is at all other times hidden. Involve your toddler in your work when possible; he can help while you do the dishes or fold laundry. Try to find time for some evening activities that the whole family can enjoy: Take a walk; you can talk with your mate while your toddler explores, and then he can fall asleep in a backpack or stroller. Go to a park or cafe where your toddler can play while you talk, and come home at bedtime. If you have older children, initiate activities they and your toddler can enjoy together, like tumbling, cooking, or drawing. Your toddler may even let you read the newspaper or mail if you do it in the bathroom while he's taking a bath, and play with him a bit now and then.

Put off nursing in the evening, if possible, until your toddler is really tired. Make sure the room is dark and quiet; you might even hang a "Do Not Disturb" sign outside the door. Remember that it's hard for your child to nurse to sleep when your muscles are taut and your breathing is fast (as you think about all the other things you think you should be doing); reading may help you relax. You may even be able to read to an older child if you keep your voice low. If nursing puts you to sleep when you want to be awake, you might ask your mate to awaken you afterward. Or get yourself ready for bed before you nurse, and enjoy your private time in the morning while your toddler sleeps on.

These measures may not bring the end of nursing any nearer, but they should reduce the number of daily nursings and give you back some control of your life. And when you're happier, you toddler probably will be, too.

THE NIGHT WAKER

Whether or not your child began sleeping through the night in infancy, as a toddler she will probably have night-waking episodes. A toddler's anxiety, fears, and anger don't disappear at night. She is prone to bad dreams, which she can't distinguish from reality. Conflicts that provoked tantrums during the day, especially in the evening, are likely to recur in your child's mind at night. A toddler may even experience night terrors—mysterious episodes of wide-eyed screaming that are entirely forgotten in the morning.

If your toddler cries frequently at night, there may be another reason besides the stress of the day's events. You'll want to consider the possibilities of a stuffy nose (from a cold or an allergy), an earache, pinworms, and teething. If the child is potty training, she may be awakening in fear of wetting the bed. Sometimes, a child may be so confused and enraged at such an awakening that she wets herself while she sits crying.

The security of an adult's arms is so important to a toddler at night that in most societies children share a bed with their parents until they are at least two or three years old (and when the children leave the parental bed it is often to sleep with other family members). A study of Hispanic West Indian families in New York found that frequent all-night bed sharing was much more common between parents and toddlers than between parents and infants. Parents in this community understood that, whereas infants could be satisfied in a crib or cradle next to the parental bed, many toddlers needed all-night bodily contact with adults (Schachter et al. 1989). Children of women who work away from home are especially likely to demand closeness with their mothers at night. Like people of all ages, toddlers rarely like to sleep alone.

Bed sharing and prolonged nursing tend to go together, both in traditional societies and in our own. It is hard, after all, to ignore a child who is trying to tear off your nightclothes. You may not hear the whimpers of a child in a room down the hall, and that child, if a heavy sleeper, may prefer just to go back to sleep rather than to yell or come find you. Still, some attentive mothers get up once, twice, or more every night for years to nurse their children back to sleep. Many of these mothers finally give in; it's easier to keep a nursing child in the parental bed. In societies where bed sharing and unrestricted nursing are the norm, children's night waking is not considered a problem.

But if you have been letting your child into your bed you may want to wean, or at least eliminate night nursing, because you're ready to bring this phase to an end. Perhaps you and your mate are feeling sex-starved. This is understandable; one study found that the more often women sleep with their babies, the less often they have sex with their mates (Cable and Rothenberger 1983). Interestingly, however, the study didn't report any complaints about the lack of sex, however, from either the women or their mates. Perhaps the familial intimacy partly makes up for the loss; one woman said that when her mate is traveling "he makes comments about how 'I feel lonely in that big bed without you guys'" (Buckley

1992). Still, you and your mate may miss having sex. Perhaps you can sneak off to another room. Or you can position yourself discreetly so that you don't awaken your child. Despite the fears of doctors, social workers, and other people, your child won't know or care what you are doing. If you have nursed her recently, she'll probably be so soundly asleep you can move about freely without disturbing her.

Overcrowding in the bed may be the most annoying part of having an "all-night" nurser. Toddlers are much bigger than they were as young infants, and many like to sleep sideways (usually with head on Mom, feet on Dad). During a bad dream, the hits and kicks can hurt if you haven't enough room to roll away. Maybe it's time to get a bigger bed, or to securely fasten a crib, if you have one, to the side of your bed.

If your child doesn't have a separate bed of her own, this may be the time to provide one, in your room or the child's own bedroom. Don't go out and buy a crib; cribs are dangerous when a child starts climbing out. A toddler can sleep safely in a bed without rails as long as it is low to the floor. A futon or an innerspring mattress works well, if the mattress sits directly on the floor or on plywood over a low frame. If the mattress is high off the floor, side rails can of course be provided, at least until your child learns not to roll off. (If she has been sleeping with you regularly, she has probably already learned this lesson.) Even if the mattress is low to the floor, you'll want to use a rug or pillows at first to cushion any falls.

If the nursery you set up while pregnant has gone unused ever since (or if you never got around to setting up a nursery), you may now want to provide your toddler not only her own bed but also her own newly decorated room, or a place in a sibling's room. A child old enough to appreciate having her own toys may like seeing them on shelves near her bed. With a night-light, perhaps, and a favorite pillow or quilt and stuffed animal toy or doll, your child may be glad to spend part of the night in her own special place.

Don't expect your child to spend all night in her new bed, though—at least not for a while. She will probably be happy to take her naps here, if you nurse her to sleep (the biggest advantage of a bed without rails is that *you* can get in and out). She may happily nurse to sleep here at night, too. If she's a heavy sleeper, she may whimper for a moment or two when it's time for her first night nursing, then fall back into a deep sleep. Congratulate yourself, as you lie awake listening from your own bed—

you've just made a big step toward weaning. Sleeping through the first night nursing may well become a pattern for her, and you yourself may soon be sleeping four to six hours without interruption. Day may be dawning before your child comes trotting in to share your bed, or calls you to hers.

If your child is a light sleeper, however, the adjustment may not happen so quickly. Your child may awaken, howling, within an hour or two of going to sleep. After several nights of this, you sensibly abandon the idea of getting your child to sleep without you. All hope is not lost, however; you can always try again a few weeks or months later. Or, if your child objects to being in a separate room, you can try moving her bed into your room, or just letting her sleep on your bedroom floor. Putting the child to bed with a willing brother or sister may also work. If your child's bedroom stands empty at night, don't feel bad. It can be a getaway for you and your mate on nights when your child or children are crowding you out of bed.

If you can't get your child to sleep without you, you can still reduce or eliminate night nursings or wean altogether while sharing a bed. You'll need to tell your child firmly that the two of you won't be nursing at night any more; you might say you're saving up the milk for the morning. Your child may be able to get back to sleep while lying against you and holding or patting your breast. Or she may prefer to lie with her back to you. You'll probably want to wear clothing that limits her access—even if you'll allow her hand in, you'll want to keep her head out.

You can try having your mate hold your child at night, but this is unlikely to work as long as you are present. Your child will probably do her best to make her father feel totally rejected; "I want Mama!" she may scream until he picks her up and dumps her in your arms. Some mothers spend several nights away from home, or at least pretend to, as a means of forcing their mates and children to adjust. One hid away in her son's room for several nights, until he learned to find comfort in his father's arms, and then she switched beds with the two of them. But such a scheme requires careful deception and an unusually cooperative mate.

However you manage the transition, you'll probably have to endure some thrashing around and tantrums as your child learns to get through the night without sucking. Once your child has adjusted, though, you may find renewed pleasure in the family bed. Cuddling with a soft, warm toddler in the night, feeling her sleepy kisses, and hearing her baby dream-talk are among the great, secret joys of family life.

THE PICKY EATER

You may be considering weaning because your breastfed toddler eats little table food, eats it irregularly, or is small for his age. If so, keep in mind that a child's growth normally slows about the beginning of his second year. As Ellyn Satter points out in *Child of Mine: Feeding with Love and Good Sense* (2000), normal growth in the second year is only one-third to one-half that of the first. The typical toddler eats erratically, skipping meals and sometimes eating next to nothing for an entire day. He can do this and thrive because of all the fat he accumulated in his first year; by burning some of this stored fat he satisfies part of his energy needs. Growing more in height than in weight, the chubby toddler transforms himself into a slender child.

Some children take virtually no foods besides breast milk until they are well into their second year. One La Leche League leader has noticed that these children tend to be late teethers; the urge to chew may develop with the ability to chew. You may wonder, though, if your child can thrive on breast milk alone. If you are well nourished and your child is gaining weight, the only nutrient he may be lacking is iron. Doctors and nutritionists once thought breastfed babies needed iron supplements from birth. This has been shown to be false; breast milk is now known to supply plenty of iron during a baby's first six months. Whether a mother can count on her milk to supply adequate iron to her twelve- or fifteen-month-old, however, is unknown. If you doubt whether your child is getting enough iron, consult your doctor for a blood test. And be patient: Your child *will* start eating soon. Stopping nursing before your child has learned to eat a variety of solids would be traumatic for him, if not dangerous to his health.

If your child is small for his age, ask yourself whether he is actually skinny, with bones showing prominently, or just plain small. Is he listless, as a chronically underfed child would be, or is he usually lively? Chances are your toddler's size is just right, for him. This is even more likely if you or your mate, or especially both of you, are short or slender. If you are both on the large side, you probably needn't worry—even within families, individuals' sizes at maturity can vary a lot. Anyway, a small toddler doesn't necessarily grow into a small adult.

If your toddler really is skinny, you should check for possible problems that may have nothing to do with nursing, such as pinworms, anemia, and a malfunctioning thyroid gland.

Whether your toddler is big or small for his age, you will want to make sure that he has plenty of opportunity to satisfy his hunger. Young children need to eat often, about once every three to four hours during the day. Meals should be quiet, relaxing times; pets, neighbor kids, and interesting toys within sight or sound of the dining table can distract a toddler from the business of eating. So can his own fatigue; if a family meal must be delayed past the toddler's naptime or bedtime, feed him early.

Eating shouldn't be a struggle for your toddler. Provide him with utensils he can manage, and let him eat with his fingers if and when he prefers. Be available to feed him when he can't or doesn't care to feed himself. Make foods easy to eat—for example, by chopping or grinding tough meat, cutting corn from the cob, skinning and cutting fruit, and mashing peas. This way you'll know he won't pass food by just because it's too difficult to eat.

What should you feed your toddler? Generally, what's good for him is probably what's good for the rest of your family—a varied diet of mostly fresh and unrefined foods. Over the course of each day, you'll want to offer fruits and vegetables, breads or grains, and protein-rich foods like meat, eggs, nuts, and beans.

As long as your toddler is nursing several times a day and you're not pregnant, he'll probably need little or no cow's milk or other dairy products (although if he isn't allergic to these it won't hurt to offer some). An omnivorous diet, however, requires some kind of drink. Unless you don't mind nursing during meals, offer water. Water should also be available between meals, whenever your toddler is thirsty. Don't make a habit of substituting juice for water; juice doesn't quench thirst as well, and drinking it frequently can lead to tooth decay and spoil the appetite for other foods. And unless juice is truly fresh or flash-frozen—not heat-treated or made from concentrate—it has lost much of the vitamin content of the original fruit.

As your toddler begins relying more on dairy milk than breast milk, make sure you provide whole milk, not low-fat or skim. Low-fat and skim milk lack the fat that a toddler needs.

Two to three cups of milk per day are all that a weaned toddler needs. As with juice, a child can get in the habit of satisfying his thirst with cow's milk, and end up drinking more than he needs. Again, encourage your toddler to satisfy his thirst with water, and treat milk as a food.

If your child is allergic to cow's milk, frequent breastfeeding is certainly the most economical alternative. If breastfeeding is coming to a close, however, you may want to provide a soy-based alternative. Commercial soy blends such as Vitasoy are good sources of protein, but most contain lesser proportions of calcium and fat than both breast milk and cow's milk. Soy-based infant formula is a better choice for a toddler. If you do buy regular soy milk, choose a brand with a high percentage of calcium (that is, one to which a lot of seaweed has been added), a larger amount of fat, and supplemental vitamin D.

The temptation to overfeed juice, milk, and other beverages is hardest to resist when bottles are allowed. If your toddler must suck at a bottle between meals, at naptime, or at bedtime, fill the bottle with water. Children who drink milk or sweet beverages from bottles all day lose their appetites for nutritious meals and snacks and also risk serious tooth decay (see "Nursing and Tooth Decay," page 144).

Don't worry about how much your toddler eats of a particular food, or even if he sometimes won't eat at all. In a famous study done in the 1920s, Clara Davis let three nine-month-olds, who had been to that point solely breastfed, begin choosing their own meals from a wide selection of natural, uncombined foods (including salt, which they occasionally ate although it made them choke and splutter). The children all tended to eat foods "in waves"—taking them in great quantities for a week or more and in moderate amounts thereafter. Still, over a six-month period, each child selected a diet that would meet with the approval of nutritionists. More important, they throve (Davis 1928).

> 66You are responsible for what your child is offered to eat, and where and when it is presented. She is responsible for how much of it she eats.99
>
> —ELLYN SATTER, *CHILD OF MINE: FEEDING WITH LOVE AND GOOD SENSE*

You can trust your toddler's instincts in the matter of diet even if you usually serve foods in combination, as soups, stews, casseroles, or the like. You will of course want to withhold any food to which your child has had an allergic reaction. Otherwise, as long as salty, sweet, or refined foods don't predominate on your family's table, your toddler should eat well there without much special attention.

Be careful, however, if your family is strictly vegetarian, that is, if you avoid eggs and dairy products as well as meat. Young children on macrobiotic, fruitarian, Rastafarian, and other diets that contain little animal foods have tended to be smaller and lighter than other children, have often showed delayed gross-motor development, and sometimes have shown delayed speech and language development (*Nutrition Reviews* 1990). In one study in well-fed Holland, weaned toddlers on macrobiotic diets got too little calories, protein, fat, calcium, riboflavin, vitamin B_{12}, and iron. Rickets, from a lack of calcium, was common among these children; so was iron-deficiency anemia. Even before weaning, the macrobiotic children may have been somewhat malnourished, since their mothers' milk was lower in both calcium and vitamin B_{12} than that of omnivorous women (Dagnelie et al. 1989).

The main problem with most strict vegetarian diets is that they are too bulky for young children—that is, children must eat great volumes of the allowed foods to get enough calories and protein, and most simply can't eat enough. Secondly, the iron and vitamin B_{12} that may be present in plant sources may not be "bio-available"—that is, usable to the body—and the high proportion of fiber in the diet may interfere with the absorption of various nutrients. These are the reasons weaning is such a dangerous passage in many poor countries. If weaning occurs before a child's digestive capacity can match his energy needs, malnutrition results. Kwashiorkor, a severe form of malnutrition, takes its name from an African word meaning "the disease of the deposed baby"—deposed, that is, by a new sibling (Riordan 1983, 318).

With some modification, however, your particular diet may be suitable for your child. You can reduce dietary fiber simply by substituting refined grains for whole grains part of the time, and you can increase caloric intake by judicious use of avocados, nut butters, and other fatty plant foods. Ellyn Satter (2000) recommends offering the vegetarian toddler plenty of foods rich in vitamin C, which helps in absorbing plant iron. Consult a nutritionist for more advice on ensuring good nutrition for your vegetarian toddler. To be on the safe side, continue nursing or feeding infant formula at least through your child's second year.

Occasionally a toddler regularly insists on nursing during meals, and shows no interest in the food on his plate. If he then nurses to sleep, it may be that he was too tired to eat, and needs his meals served a little earlier. Or maybe he nurses at mealtimes because he is hungry, and hasn't yet learned to associate table food with appetite satisfaction; again, dinner should be served *before* he is desperate for the breast. Or, if a toddler tries to get your attention all through dinner preparations, maybe he needs time at the breast before you start making dinner. In the last case, he'll probably have his appetite back by the time dinner is ready, which will likely be sooner than it would be if you kept putting him off. If necessary, you can tell your toddler that you won't be nursing him during meals anymore, and that he'll have to wait until later.

Finally, take advantage of your toddler's natural curiosity by making eating an adventure. If you feed your toddler on little but beans and tortillas, he may eat little else until he's a teenager. Any foods you'll expect him to eat in childhood you should introduce now, not after he turns three and becomes much more conservative. Involve your toddler in shopping for and preparing what he eats. Let him eat peas, strawberries, cherry tomatoes, and the like directly from the garden, if you have one. Don't insist on cooking foods that would be just as healthful and prettier served raw. Try cutting foods various ways—occasionally, perhaps, in fanciful shapes. Pay attention when he begins telling you what shapes he prefers. If eating is pleasurable as well as healthful for you, your toddler will probably experience it the same way.

THE AGGRESSIVE TODDLER

A toddler's mobility, curiosity, and frequent frustrations all affect the way she nurses. For the mother, the resulting behavior may cause annoyance, pain, and a desire to end nursing as soon as possible.

A toddler may seek solace from her frustrations by nursing hard and long, perhaps for more hours per day than she nursed as a newborn. It may help to nurse her in a quiet place without distractions, where she may more quickly relax and, possibly, get to sleep. You might also ask yourself what circumstances are causing her frustrations—is her sister, for instance, continually taking toys away from her?—and then make whatever changes you can to prevent these occurrences. If necessary for your own comfort, you might also restrict the number or length of nursings.

Most toddlers enjoy acrobatic nursing—trying out as many positions as possible while still keeping hold of the nipple. A mother may find these antics amusing at times, but they can also be annoying and even painful. Unless a toddler is well positioned for nursing, friction from her sharp little teeth may cause injury to the nipple. And if she slips or falls while the nipple is in her mouth, she may hurt her mother as well as herself. Encourage your child to get her playing over with before nursing, and then to settle down into a comfortable position before you suckle her.

A nursing toddler may treat the breast she isn't sucking, or her mother's entire body, as a plaything or even as a punching bag. She may paw at the breast, twiddle or pinch the nipple, play with her mother's hair, poke at her belly button, or stick her fingers in her mother's mouth, eyes, or nose. She may slap, pummel, and kick. It's a good idea to try to stop such behavior before it becomes habitual. Many toddlers, however, insist on keeping the "free hand," as Norma Jane Bumgarner (1982) calls it, on the mother's free breast. Most commonly, they twiddle the nipple. You might discourage this by wearing clothes that are hard to pull up, or by offering something else for your child to fiddle with, such as a small stuffed toy. Or you might explain that you don't like it when your child plays with your nipple, but that she may pat or hold your breast. Putting your hand over your child's may help keep it still. Many mothers just learn to ignore the twiddling.

Weaning won't necessarily end annoying habits like hair pulling and mouth poking. A one-year-old's aggressiveness might best be seen as a developmental step beyond the passive fulfillment of infancy. Even if weaning changes the way a toddler's aggression is expressed, the aggression won't just disappear. A mother who persists in nursing through this stage will find aggressiveness gradually replaced by a desire to please, expressed in nursing by gentle holding and caressing, and a willingness to comply with the mother's requests.

THE SENSUOUS TODDLER

A woman may decide to wean upon realizing what a sensuous experience nursing is, for both her child and herself. But the sensuous aspect of breastfeeding should have been obvious from the start. Both mother and baby take pleasure in the smells of each other's bodies, the feel of each other's skin, the hardening and softening of the breast as the milk lets down and is sucked out, the shared looks. Most nursing mothers frequently stroke and kiss their babies. Nursing is more than feeding; it is an act of love. This is one reason many people are embarrassed in the presence of a nursing couple: The flushed cheeks, loving touches, and contented smiles can make the outsider feel witness to an intimate encounter.

Oxytocin, the hormone produced when milk lets down, is also produced during lovemaking. Some people call oxytocin "the hormone of love."

As a baby grows into a toddler, he becomes a more active participant in this love affair. The mother, and not just the breast, becomes the child's love object. While nursing he may ceaselessly paw her—until, eventually, he learns to stroke tenderly. Stroking his mother may even become more important to the child than sucking at her breasts. He may insist that both breasts be fully exposed while he nurses, and he may want to strip off his clothes. When nursing naked he will probably explore his genitals, and he may have an erection. Although we are using male pronouns here, a female toddler will behave in much the same way.

A mother may worry because her child's sucking and caresses make *her* feel sexually aroused. Feelings of sexual arousal can't necessarily be suppressed just because the stimulation comes from a baby or toddler. But having these feelings doesn't make a mother attempt to have some sort of genital sex with her child. Mothers just don't do that. Nursing may, however, be a frequent prelude to sex with a mate.

Nursing mothers in our society may have trouble accepting sexual feelings—their children's and their own—as natural and good. Even if you disdain the notion that children are born sinful, you probably know plenty of people who believe that whatever comes naturally is evil, uncivilized, or at best suspicious. Some social workers view "prolonged" nursing and bed sharing as indicators of child abuse. What if such people, you may wonder, found out about *your* relationship with your child?

Your child's sensuality is perfectly normal. You may, however, want to place some limits on his sensual expression. If you're uncomfortable with your toddler's fondling his genitals, make sure he is dressed in a diaper or underpants, or more, before you nurse him. You might allow him to pat but not stroke your breasts, or else request that he keep his hand still, and help him comply by holding his hand. You might try offering something else smooth or soft to stroke, such as a piece of satin fabric. If your child is embarrassing you by exposing your breasts in public, you might decide to nurse him only at home in the future. It is generally easier to keep a nursing relationship private than to stop nursing altogether.

Letting your child caress you now may even help in weaning a little later. If stroking becomes more important to your child than sucking, he may agree to give up nursing if he can still touch your breasts. Letting him put his hand down your shirt, even for a few moments, may allow him to calm down or go back to sleep without nursing at all. Many children continue to find quick comfort this way, when they're upset, for months after weaning.

NURSING AND TOOTH DECAY

You may be considering weaning your toddler because she has "bottle-mouth, " "baby-bottle tooth decay," or "nursing caries." These are among the various terms used to refer to a pattern of serious dental decay, especially of the top front teeth, that begins in infancy. The affected teeth are those that erupt early and are unprotected by the tongue during suckling. First appearing as brown or black spots on the front, back, or sides of the teeth, nursing caries have become common among bottle-fed babies, many of whom drink real or artificial fruit juices, soda, or milk throughout the day. The sugars in these drinks feed bacteria that produce acid, which decays tooth enamel; the acid in juices, additionally, erodes the enamel directly. Nursing caries are especially common among children who take bottles to bed—not just bottles of juice or other sweet beverages, but even bottles of formula or milk. During sleep the milk drips from the bottle and pools in the mouth, where bacteria ferment the milk sugar (lactose) into acid that demineralize the teeth.

Nursing caries sometimes appear among breastfed children. When this happens, a dentist may blame the problem on breastfeeding, especially nighttime breastfeeding, since during sleep the flow of saliva is diminished, and saliva contains an enzyme that protects against dental disease. In recent years scientists have firmly established, however, that breastfeeding doesn't cause tooth decay. Because the flow of milk from a mother's nipple occurs far back in the mouth and is controlled by the baby's sucking, the milk is swallowed, reflexively, before it can pool in the mouth. And, unlike milk from a bottle, breast milk doesn't drip into the mouth after a baby stops sucking. Besides, whereas formula is cariogenic—that is, it causes cavities—breast milk, by itself, is not; in fact, it can actually build enamel by depositing calcium and phosphorus on the teeth (Sheikh and Erickson 1996, Erickson and Mazhari 1999). In isolated nonindustrial societies in which children are nursed day and night for two or more years, dental decay among children is very rare. When refined sugar is introduced into the diet, however, tooth decay becomes commonplace.

There are many reasons that a breastfed toddler might tend to develop dental caries. Since a baby's teeth begin forming in the womb, their resistance to decay depends partially on how well they mineralize during pregnancy. A mother's fever, illness, antibiotic medication, or malnourishment during pregnancy can disrupt this mineralization. High fevers in a baby before the teeth erupt can also interrupt mineralization; so can a premature birth. Food allergies and respiratory infections can lead to tooth decay, because if a child is perpetually congested he may breathe through his mouth, thus drying up the saliva, which normally protects the teeth. Lead exposure, through water, breast milk, or ingested paint, also seems to cause cavities, either by stunting the development of the saliva glands or by hindering enamel growth (Watson et al. 1997). A child may also have a genetic susceptibility to tooth decay or poor enamel formation.

In both breast- and bottle-fed children, the biggest contributor to tooth decay is sugary foods. Scientists are currently arguing over whether raisins and other sticky dried fruits do children's teeth more harm than good, but none doubt that the refined sugars (including corn syrup) in packaged drinks, breakfast cereals, baked goods, and desserts contribute to tooth decay in many toddlers. Oral bacteria multiply the most when sweets are eaten frequently or constantly—for example, when a child sucks on a hard candy, snacks continually from a little bag of breakfast cereal, or carries around a bottle of sweetened juice.

For tooth decay to occur, certain bacteria must be present in the mouth. The most common microorganism responsible for caries on the crowns of the teeth is *Streptococcus mutans* (this is not the same microorganism responsible for strep throat). Most five-year-olds have *S. mutans* in their mouths, as do older people, but few one-year-olds do. Toddlers with rampant nursing caries, however, have one hundred times more of this bacteria in their mouths than do toddlers without tooth decay (Matee et al. 1993). In babies with *S. mutans*, the microorganism has usually been transmitted from the mother or mate, or someone else in the family, through saliva. Sharing food and utensils and even kissing can enable *S. mutans* to travel from one mouth to another. Some parents have reduced their strep counts, making themselves less infective to their children, by limiting sugary foods and maintaining good dental hygiene (Ripa 1988).

With your help, your toddler can practice dental hygiene, too. The American Academy of Pediatric Dentistry recommends cleaning a baby's mouth *from birth* with a soft infant toothbrush and water. Easier said than done! Most parents wait until the teeth begin to erupt, and begin with a soft, damp cloth rather than a toothbrush. A bedtime cleaning is most important. Introduce a small, soft toothbrush when you can, and brush your child's teeth for him until he is able to do it well himself. If your water supply isn't fluoridated, you may already be giving your child a fluoride supplement. If not, ask your child's dentist or doctor about a prescription.

If nursing caries are detected early enough, they may be treated in the dentist's office, sometimes without even local anesthesia, if the child is able to cooperate. The cavities in front may be filled with tooth-colored "composite," a plastic material that is bonded to the teeth. Treatment can sometimes be postponed until the child is older, if the condition is monitored and the teeth are well cared for, perhaps with topical fluoride treatments as well as brushing and good dietary habits. Advanced decay, however, may necessitate prompt treatment that a toddler can't sit still through. In such a case, general anesthesia or sedatives are administered, usually in the hospital. The decayed teeth may be capped, or, if necessary, extracted.

If you suspect your child has decayed teeth, do have your child examined soon. A dentist's diagnosis of nursing caries would certainly indicate that you should evaluate your child's diet and dental hygiene, and your own as well. Have your water and any flaking paint in your house tested for lead (and keep in mind that the calcium in breast milk can reduce lead absorption in a nursing child's gastrointestinal tract). If the dentist insists that you wean immediately and you and your child aren't ready, get another opinion. Given the many benefits of nursing for both mother and toddler, no amount of dental decay is a reason to wean completely.

How to Wean Your Toddler

Writers on breastfeeding have grouped weaning methods under two categories, gradual weaning and abrupt weaning. At least one writer uses the term *traumatic weaning* synonymously with *abrupt weaning,* to foster the idea that abrupt weaning is always traumatic. But gradual weaning can also be traumatic, if not in the sense that it causes permanent psychic damage, then at least in that it can make a child anxious for a period of weeks or months. Carried out with empathy, resolve, and planning, weaning of either sort should cause a child no irreparable harm.

WEANING GRADUALLY

This is our culturally approved way of weaning. It's supposed to happen like this: When the child loses interest in a particular daily feeding, you begin skipping that feeding. You don't refuse the breast, you just instead offer a bottle or cup, depending on the child's age and your own preference. Every week or so you replace another breastfeeding with a bottle or cup, until your milk is gone and nursing is over.

This paradigm, which presumes that your child is on some sort of feeding schedule and that her only motive to nurse is hunger, is hard to apply to a child who nurses whenever she feels like it, especially if she nurses over a dozen times a day. Besides, the paradigm ignores the fact that, for a toddler, nursing is a tool for self-soothing and relaxation, and a source of pure pleasure.

Another version of gradual weaning, summed up in the slogan "Don't offer, don't refuse," prescribes child-led, not mother-led, weaning. Children normally take an active role in the weaning process, by eating more and more table foods and gradually demanding less time at the breast. But few children stop nursing altogether before the age of three or four unless they get plenty of encouragement. To many women, "Don't offer, don't refuse" means, in practice, "Don't wean."

For women who want to stop nursing while their children are still toddlers, Norma Jane Bumgarner (2000) and other writers have identified several techniques for gradual weaning, including distraction, substitution, postponement, and shortened nursings. Children nearing three years of age may also accept weaning through bargaining (see Chapter 5). We've already discussed some ways gradual weaning techniques might be applied in problem situations, but here we'll address the techniques specifically.

Shortened Nursings

Some mothers are able to reduce the time they spend nursing by saying, "OK, you can nurse for just a minute," and then counting out loud or using a watch to count down the seconds. Other women allow only as much time as it takes them to sing the alphabet (an extra benefit is that the child learns her ABCs).

Some children can be satisfied with very brief nursings; one even initiated the practice of "nursie for second," which meant she briefly put her mouth on the breast (Owen 1989, 51-52). Many children, however, would be devastated to have to end a nursing just after having begun it. Timing nursings might work best when a child seems to want just a bit of reassurance rather than a meal or a nap.

Even if your child resents any clocking of her time at the breast, you might be able to cut a nursing short by distracting her—for instance, by grabbing a picture book, offering lunch, or starting a game of "This Little Piggie." A handy doll or puppet might be especially effective in talking your child into another activity.

Postponement

"I'll nurse you as soon as I finish making this sandwich," you might say, and your two-year-old might sit quietly in a high chair beside you until you finish. If you're nursing only occasionally during the afternoon or evening, you might be able to stop altogether by saying, "Let's save up the milk for bedtime." Or you might be able to stop middle-of-the-night feedings by saying, "Let's save up the milk till morning."

Postponing nursing gets easier the older a child gets. But don't expect it to work well with most children under two. Of course you'll postpone some nursings with a one-year-old, out of necessity, but your child may scream until you finish making that sandwich. This is OK, as long

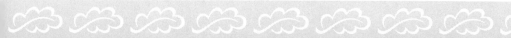

as you keep your word. Your child will eventually learn that gratification *can* be delayed. Do try to be precise about what you've got to do before nursing. "I'll come in a little while," or even "Just wait ten minutes," has little meaning for a toddler.

It helps to make a clear rule for your child to follow: "We can nurse only when it's dark outside," for example, or "We can nurse only when we're at home." If you try this, set only one rule at a time, keep it simple, and apply it consistently.

Substitution

Toddlers often nurse because they're hungry or—especially in hot weather—thirsty. One mother we know was able to wean her toddler just by offering food or a drink whenever the child wanted to nurse. Substitution is more likely to be effective, however, if you anticipate your child's needs: Have food or drink ready before he feels the urge to nurse. Serve a meal or snack every few hours, and provide a drink with meals. You might also keep a water dispenser and special cup accessible to your toddler (if you do, of course, expect some spills).

If you're not a morning person, providing a substitute for your child's first morning nursing may be difficult. One woman managed to rouse herself enough to set out a bowl of cereal and milk; then she went back to bed and slept while her child ate. Some women get their mates to help in the morning. "He would give her breakfast and after breakfast I would join them," said one mother. "I hid out in my bedroom in the mornings for about a week" (Owen 1989, 14-15).

You may or may not be comfortable providing substitutes for your child's sucking needs. Some children do start sucking on thumbs, fingers, bottles, or pacifiers during weaning, and many of these children keep up the habit for years. Some parents see no harm in this, although they must pay extra attention to sanitation and, if bottles are used, to the danger of "juice abuse." A child who falls while sucking at a bottle may injure his mouth, and if he takes a bottle to bed he risks serious tooth decay. At some point, too, a child weaned to a bottle or pacifier must be weaned *from* the dummy nipple. Some parents find thumb-sucking embarrassing, but it is relatively harmless provided it doesn't continue so long that it causes orthodontic damage.

A mother and her child may find substitutes, too, for the comfort and pleasure nursing provides. Some children transfer their feelings to so-called transitional objects, like blankets, stuffed toy animals, and sometimes even Mama's satin underclothes. Others start watching a lot of television. Such a dependence may be short-lived, or it may continue for years. Many parents, again, see no harm in using such things, but others worry about the psychic consequences of a strong early attachment to inanimate objects. Others worry in particular about the effects of television's confusing visual images on a very young mind. Doctors worry, too; the American Academy of Pediatrics advises against *any* television watching for children under two years.

Some children insist on a physical attachment to their mothers, but will let it take an alternative form. For toddlers, staying close to Mama is usually more important than having her milk or sucking. A toddler may spend a lot of time holding her mother's breast, or may reach for it whenever she is tired or when strangers are around. Or she may clutch her mother's hair in her fist, perhaps tugging a bit when she feels insecure. If a new baby comes between mother and toddler, even holding hands (over or around the baby) may make nights easier. Weaning may go a lot smoother if a mother can placidly accept such expressions of attachment.

An immaterial substitute for nursing was suggested by a follower of Rudolf Steiner: "You don't have to give up nursing completely," she told her two-year-old. "You can still nurse in your dreams." Since the family had spent much time discussing dreams and their importance, this satisfied him. He went to sleep eagerly from then on, his mother said, and slept more soundly than before.

Distraction

This is the most time-consuming technique of gradual weaning, but along with substitution it is also the most effective. You distract a toddler from nursing by making life so interesting he doesn't even think about the breast. You read him books, help him ride his trike, sing to him, rock him, tickle him, tumble with him, invite other kids to visit him, and take him on walks, picnics, and other outings. One toddler gave up nursing during a camping trip; he "had such wonderful full days," his mother said, "he didn't need to nurse" (Owen 1989, 15).

Family members and friends can often distract a toddler from wanting to nurse. One mother took her sister along to a week-long business convention so the sister could care for the children while the mother attended cocktail parties and dinners. With his beloved aunt taking him on adventures all over the city, the toddler forgot about nursing.

If your toddler isn't crazy about her aunt, however, or if she isn't the outgoing sort, this weaning strategy won't work. When a child needs to be close to Mama most of the time, *Mama* must provide the distractions.

If your child is shy, exciting places like a convention center (or a zoo, amusement park, or shopping mall) may serve not to distract the child but to make her want to nurse more. Some children nurse as a way of retreating from threatening situations. On a trip overseas, one shy toddler not only started nursing more, she also broke out in hives (Owen 1989, 14). She weaned later without much difficulty, in the peace and quiet of her own home.

Many women find spring and summer the best times to wean because these seasons offer so many distractions—walks in the sun, trips to the pool, park and beach visits, swarming insects and neighborhood children, good times in the sandbox. Your toddler may nurse much less when long days and warm weather keep you both outdoors most of the time. At night, while looking at the stars and listening to the crickets, a toddler may fall peacefully asleep or at least stop her crying.

Unfortunately, most mothers need to spend a lot of time indoors, cleaning, cooking, and doing desk work. Enlist your child's help with the housework when you can (this will slow you down, of course, but you'll get something done besides nursing). An "emergency" toy basket can come in handy when you need to think, write, or carry on an important telephone conversation. If your child wants to be held, carry her in a backpack. Let her fall asleep as you run errands. Stay on your feet except when you're ready to play or work with your child, and then sit on the floor instead of on a couch or in a comfy armchair—unless you are prepared with a picture book in your hands.

Books are a favorite distraction from the breast. For a child under two, choose simple stories that are understandable from the pictures alone. Your child may like hearing a rhythmic, repetitious text, or she may prefer just to turn the pages and look at the pictures. As the two of

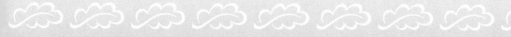

you point and exclaim, your toddler learns to concentrate, to compre-hend, and to express herself. Cuddled in your lap, she also learns to asso-ciate books with comfort. Over time the two of you will set a pattern: Your child will probably find both solace and stimulation in books for the rest of her life.

Particular books may even address how your child is feeling about weaning. *Maggie's Weaning,* by Mary Joan Deutschbein, is about a tod-dler who watches a new baby being nursed and remembers when she was nursed and weaned. *Michele: The Nursing Toddler,* by Jane M. Pinczuk, only hints that nursing will end for Michele; the book concludes, "One thing Michele always knew—she'll still have lots of love when her nurs-ing days are through."

Because the bedtime nursing is often the hardest to give up, new bed-time rituals are an important form of distraction. In addition to books, back rubs, storytelling, singing and rocking, and exchanging hugs and kisses may soothe a child to sleep. If you incorporate some of these ac-tivities into your nightly routine while still nursing, weaning will be eas-ier, since your child will be losing only one part of a loving evening ritual.

A child's father may be able to take over at bedtime—or he may not, as long as the mother is in the house. Some women go out in the evenings until the new bedtime ritual is established. But if your child is already feeling anxious, about weaning or anything else, your nights out can feel to her like abandonment. One toddler slept on top of her mother's face, clutching her hair, after the mother went out two evenings in a row. A toddler may much prefer bedtime without the breast over bedtime with-out Mama.

Weaning an avid nurser by distraction requires a lot of diligence. You can't let your child see you undressed. You may have to avoid cradling your child in your arms, or even sitting or lying down in her presence. You may have to stay away from favorite nursing places, such as the bed or couch, or move the favorite nursing chair into another room. You may have to avoid doing things that prompted nursing before, such as talking on the phone.

FAVORITE DISTRACTIONS FOR TODDLERS	
Books	Games
Outings	Back rubs
Water	Other kids
Toys	Dad

When Gradual Weaning Isn't Working

It can be nearly impossible for a woman to carry on with her daily life while keeping her child from thinking about nursing. For this reason she may have trouble being consistent: Sometimes she may succeed with distractions and substitutions, but often she may be preoccupied and so end up nursing most of the day, and other times she may just get fed up and say no. Her difficulties are compounded if, besides feeling tired of nursing, she also feels guilty over denying her toddler what the child loves best, or if she isn't quite ready to give up the nursing relationship herself. The child senses her mother's displeasure, confusion, or both, feels anxious, and so demands to nurse more to allay her own anxiety. One child called nursing *why,* as in "Why can't I have some?" (Owen 1989, 13). Another, who had been potty-trained, reverted to wearing diapers. Her mother explained, "To me I was playing the bad guy, and the whole thing was a total disaster" (Owen 1989, 61). Many children become clingy and fretful during gradual weaning.

Fretfulness, of course, may have causes other than weaning. Colds, flus, ear infections, teething, injuries, and emotional upsets can all increase a child's need for the breast. If you can't meet your child's needs through substitute forms of attention, consider what else is going on in your child's life, and think about taking a break from your weaning efforts. You can always try again when your child is feeling better.

Some women give up trying to wean their toddlers; they wait until the children near three years and become easier to reason with. Other women can't wait. They may simply be tired of nursing; they may believe the child is too old to nurse; they may think an upcoming separation will be easier if the child is weaned; or they may face pressure to wean

from mates, relatives, or friends. And so they try to put a quick end to nursing.

WEANING ABRUPTLY

In many societies, abrupt weaning is the norm, occurring at a culturally prescribed time. This doesn't mean that a child is totally breastfed one day and on an adult diet the next. Generally, children weaned suddenly are at least two years old and eating a variety of foods. In Western society today, women who wean suddenly often do so because of an unavoidable separation from their children or a need for dangerous drugs, such as chemotherapy. Some women, however, wean abruptly on impulse.

The Aversion Method

This can include as many as three techniques, involving the taste and appearance of the breast and the mother's strong words. A native of Mexico remembered her mother using all three techniques to wean her three children. The mother rubbed her breasts with unsweetened cocoa powder and told the children it was feces; most of them, understandably, wouldn't even taste the "caca." The Arapesh of New Guinea weaned children the same way, using mud instead of cocoa and "every strongly pantomimed expression of disgust," although they did this only when a mother became pregnant before her older child turned three or four (Mead 1963, 38).

Appearance alone may sometimes scare a child away from the breast forever. In *A Tree Grows in Brooklyn,* Betty Smith (1943) writes of a mother who weaned her six-year-old by blackening one breast with stove polish, then drawing with lipstick "a wide ugly mouth with frightening teeth in the vicinity of the nipple." After hiding under the bed for twenty-four hours, the boy "went back to drinking black coffee." We imagine most children would be more amused than frightened by Mama's painting a monstrous face on her breast, but the story may be based on a real incident.

A mother's words alone can also put an end to nursing. A Malian woman reportedly told her child that her milk "had turned bad because there were worms in her breast." The child did not try to nurse again (Dettwyler 1987).

Fortunately, perhaps, most women who use the aversion method rely more on distaste than fear. In societies all over the world, women have weaned their toddlers by daubing bitter or peppery substances on their breasts, including aloe, quinine, hot pepper, soot, wormwood, mustard, and bile. Although painting the breasts with bitter substances apparently became less common in the West after the mid-eighteenth century, this may be because children after this time were generally weaned in the first year after birth (Fildes 1986, 377). Infants, if not less attached to the breast than toddlers, are certainly less able to fight for it. Although abrupt weaning of any sort is condemned by most writers on children's health—and has been condemned by such persons for centuries—some contemporary American women do admit applying distasteful substances to their breasts to discourage nursing, and many of these women claim success. Two used an herbal mixture concocted for a poison-oak rash; their children, they report, said, "Yuck," and refused to nurse again (Owen 1989, 57).

Although these children reportedly gave up nursing immediately with no sign of anxiety, others are more determined to continue. One mother we know tried to discourage her two-year-old, Tim, by applying to her breasts, at various times, aloe vera, cocoa powder, prepared mustard, hot mustard powder, Angostura bitters, and, finally, Stopzit, a commercial product meant for discouraging nail-biting and thumb-sucking. Her son responded with only mild complaints and grimaces until she applied the Stopzit, whose extremely bitter taste lasts for several hours. With Stopzit she was able to greatly reduce the number of daily nursings—until she ran out of the stuff, at which point her son resumed nursing as much as ever.

Even when foul-tasting substances are effective in weaning, they may be unsafe for a nursing child, especially if they are repeatedly licked off. Hot pepper can burn painfully. Aloe vera is a laxative, mustard an emetic. Cocoa contains caffeine, and some children are allergic to chocolate in all forms. Most bitter plant substances, actually, may be at least mildly toxic to humans. Whether these substances are dangerous to a nursing child may depend on how quickly the child gives up the breast.

Applying nasty substances to the breast may have emotional as well as physical effects. Zulu children, according to one study, would watch, apparently bewildered or frightened, while their mothers smeared aloe on their breasts. The children usually weaned quickly, often without attempting to nurse even once more, but the mother-child relationship was for several weeks quite disturbed: A child would go through stages of alternately attacking and ignoring her mother, acting fretful and clingy, and showing unusual independence. Destructive behavior was common in the weeks after weaning, as were intense tantrums and sleep problems. Although most of these effects were short-lived, children weaned earlier than usual (at about fifteen months rather than eighteen) became especially aggressive and remained disturbed much longer. And most Zulu children remained somewhat alienated from or ambivalent about their mothers, and more aggressive generally (Albino and Thompson 1956).

A child may be spared a sense of betrayal if her mother successfully hides the cause of the bad taste on her breast. One of the women who used the poison-oak remedy didn't let her child see her apply the mixture, which was apparently invisible. Although the child "thrashed around a bit" the first night, she seemed to experience no anger and little anxiety about weaning; she apparently assumed that the milk, or the breast, had just stopped tasting good (Owen 1989, 58).

But if a child keeps nursing in spite of the bad taste, the substance may have to be applied quite often, and the more often the mother applies it the more likely that the child will suspect deceit. Tim, whose mother tried a variety of substances, must have been suspicious, especially since some of the substances were quite visible on the skin. His mother described him as very clingy and fussy during the several weeks she tried to wean him by aversion, after which she resumed nursing at his will. During these weeks of attempted weaning, Tim wanted nothing to do with his father, and at day care he frequently pointed to his open mouth, said "Mama," and shook his head sadly. Tim weaned easily two months later, after an eleven-day separation from his mother.

A child close to three years old may be less upset by his mother's efforts to wean by aversion, but also better able to circumvent these efforts. A graduate student from Nepal remembered that, after his mother applied something bitter to her nipples, he collected saliva in his mouth, took a few wet sucks, spit out the bitter substance, and resumed nursing. His mother gave up the technique (Berg 1994).

The Separation Method

Tim's mother tried to wean her child before a planned separation so that he wouldn't miss her as much. Other women plan prolonged separations from their children as a way of accomplishing weaning. Weaning by separation was common in pre-industrial England, and it was the favored weaning method in the American colonies (Fildes 1986, 379). It is widely used today in non-Western societies, often to complete the weaning process after a period of minimal breastfeeding. Some Western mothers wean this way, too. A mother leaves her child with the father, or sends the child to stay with grandparents, other relatives, or friends, for several days or longer.

Writers on children's health and parenting have long condemned weaning by separation. A young child has little sense of time, they say, so when Mama goes away for more than a day or two he may feel she is gone for good, and may begin mourning her. The sudden withdrawal of both the comfort of the breast and the security of his mother's presence can be overwhelming for a toddler.

Valerie Fildes (1986, 380) suggests that weaning by separation could have caused the prevalence of melancholia in late sixteenth- and seventeenth-century England. Melancholia was an upper-class complaint, and upper-class children often suffered a particularly harsh sort of separation. Sent out as young infants to wet nurses, they left their foster mothers forever at weaning, to join unfamiliar families in unfamiliar homes. For these children, "Mama" never came back.

The children we know of who were weaned by separation certainly missed their mothers while they were gone, but seemed to experience no long-term sadness. Tim cried for four hours on his second night without his mother, and wouldn't let his grandmother touch him for a week, although he was affectionate with his grandfather. After Tim's reunion with his mother he wanted to resume nursing, but accepted her refusal

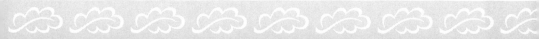

with minimal fuss; he acted neither detached nor clingy. He was "his happy, easygoing self," his mother said. Like other women with similar experiences, Tim's mother felt weaning by separation was relatively easy; she regretted the long, anxious weeks of trying—and failing—to wean before her trip.

If you must be separated from your nursing toddler for a number of days or weeks, do leave him with loved ones—including any siblings, if possible. Provide plenty of familiar objects—a blanket or pillow, a stuffed animal or doll, a music box, a picture of yourself. Before the separation, try to give your child a sense of how long it will last; counting nights may make more sense to him than counting days. Tell the caregivers about your child's favorite foods and activities, and whatever ways have worked in the past to get him to sleep without nursing. If your child is used to nursing during the night, make sure the caregivers are prepared for a rough night or two. They will probably need to tell your child, perhaps several times a day, that Mama will be back soon.

If the separation lasts less than two or three weeks, don't expect to come back to a child "well weaned," as a seventeenth-century father put it (Fildes 1986, 379). Although your child may not try to nurse for a day or so, he will probably still remember the pleasure of nursing, and how to nurse. When the two of you get back to most of your old routines, he may expect to resume nursing as well.

You may still have milk, too, especially if you expressed milk during the separation. If you don't mind resuming nursing, go ahead—your milk supply will probably increase again to meet your child's needs. You need not nurse as much as before the separation, however, if you don't wish to. If your child is out of the habit of sucking for comfort or attention throughout the day and night, he may need to nurse only once or twice in twenty-four hours, such as at bedtime and in the early morning.

If you don't want to resume nursing after a separation, this may be a good time to "just say no." If the separation lasted a week or more, your child should be much less attached to the breast than previously, and you should be over any engorgement. If your milk isn't "dried up," the supply will probably soon be negligible. Your toddler may accept your excuse that "the milk's all gone," and may go to sleep with a story instead of the breast. After a few days or weeks of occasional clinginess and tantrums, your child may truly be well weaned.

Just Saying No

Some women wean abruptly without either leaving their children or using aversion techniques. A woman may wean this way on doctor's orders, because of a drug she is taking or an illness she has, or she may do it on dentists' orders, because her child has nursing caries. Or she may decide on her own—often impulsively—to suddenly stop nursing. Explained Omar's mother, "I just said one day, 'I've had it! I don't want to do this anymore'" (Owen 1989, 44).

A mother who suddenly decides to stop nursing may have tried gradual weaning methods for many months, with little or no success. If her child is a nonstop nurser, she may be at her wits' end when she decides to quit, as was Karen, whose son Adam would suck for an hour at a time. One day, after twice nursing him to sleep only to have him awaken and demand more just as she got up from the bed, Karen "said, 'No more, period! . . . I was at a point where there were a lot more things I wanted to do. That's it—I'm done! I hadn't planned it'" (Owen 1989, 35-36).

Since a child weaned in this way knows that the milk is still available and tasty, the mother must be very firm in her refusal to nurse. The child will have an easier time if nursings are down to a few a day before they stop altogether, if the mother can give a good reason for denying the breast, and if she provides a lot of extra comforting for several days or weeks. She may need to put a great deal of energy into providing substitutes and distractions. Even if she doesn't, though, a sudden weaning isn't necessarily traumatic. Whereas Adam "fussed for two weeks," Omar, said his mother, just took the cup whenever she gave it to him (Owen 1989, 36, 44).

If you wean abruptly, by any technique, you risk getting painfully engorged and possibly coming down with a breast infection. Make sure you express just enough milk to keep yourself comfortable, and wear a supportive bra. Ice packs and mild pain relievers can help, too, as can sage tea (see page 67).

WEANING GENTLY

Child-care "experts" in our society virtually all recommend gradual weaning, and some use the term *gentle weaning* to mean the same thing.

As we've shown, however, gradual weaning sometimes induces prolonged anxiety in a child or augments anxiety arising from other causes. In such a case it can hardly be considered gentle. For us, weaning gently means weaning with empathy. It means understanding your child's particular needs and feelings, and also your own. Gentle weaning is usually slow and relatively late, but not always. It generally occurs after a child is eating and drinking other foods well, when she is healthy and free from major stresses, and when family life is stable. Gentle weaning happens without nagging and complaining. It includes substitutes for the breast—like the rich and tasty foods given to weanlings in many societies, and the picture books that probably clutter your home. Your toddler knows that if she can get you to look at some of those books with her, she'll have your full attention for a while, and some bodily contact with you, too. Weaning gently means staying close to your child, and providing at least as much affectionate contact as you did before weaning.

Don't try to wean your toddler during times of stress—for example, just before or after a move, during toilet training, or soon after bringing home a new puppy.

Gentle weaning is carried out with resolve, for a mother's own confidence goes far in allaying a child's anxiety. Setting clear limits and sticking to them keeps your child from wearing herself out in trying to break your resolve, over and over again.

But gentle weaning also requires flexibility. If your efforts to wean are making your child very anxious, and if you *can* continue nursing for a while (if only once or twice a day), it's best to change your plans. If you do, your child will probably soon be her happy self, and may wean with much less distress in a few months' time.

Gentle weaning may involve explanations. If you're pregnant and suffering from sore nipples, why not say so? "I just treated him as if he were a smart person," one mother said of her not-yet-two-year-old (Owen 1989, 41). Children try hard to cooperate when their parents really need their help. Your child may even get the idea that it was *her* idea to wean, as did Sequoia, whose mother got numerous breast infections while nursing both Sequoia and a newborn. "I stopped by myself so you won't get a breast infection," Sequoia said (Owen 1989, 81).

Gentle weaning means not trying to rush a child's development unnecessarily. It may be true that weaning sometimes promotes development in other areas, like talking and using the potty. But, no matter when you wean, your child *will* learn to speak clearly and use the toilet in time, even if you provide little or no direct encouragement. And, whether or not you work at weaning, she *will* learn to do without the breast. She may well cling to some baby ways for years: Some otherwise normal children wet the bed at five, some suck their thumbs when they are seven, and some fail to pronounce *l*'s and *r*'s when they are ten. Weaning long before your child is ready will only force her to find some other way of satisfying her infantile needs. She may actually regress in some areas, by needing diapers again, perhaps, or taking up thumb-sucking. So work on changing behavior you can't stand, at the breast or otherwise, and try to be patient with everything else. Above all, avoid comparing your child with others you know. All children grow up eventually!

five

WEANING YOUR CHILD OVER THREE

EYOND A CHILD'S THIRD YEAR, both nursing and weaning are usually little trouble. Most children this age nurse only once or twice a day, if that often. Many prefer to nurse in privacy, and those who want to nurse at awkward times or in inconvenient places will usually agree to wait a while, without fuss, at a mother's request. The child over three can usually get to sleep without trouble when her mother is away for the evening or even for an entire day or two. And the child past three generally gives up nursing easily—though not necessarily voluntarily.

Like many mothers of nursing children over three, though, you may feel anxious about your nursing relationship, or eager to stop nursing and unsure how to go about it. Your mate may want your child out of your bed, or you may feel that you'll all sleep better if night nursings, or all nursings, stop. If your three-, four- or five-year-old nurses many times during the day or night or both, you may feel she controls the nursing relationship at your expense. Perhaps you see your child as just too big and grown-up to nurse. You may feel restless, as if you're stuck in one phase of child-rearing long after the mothers of your child's peers have moved on to the next. Maybe you need the sense of completion that weaning can bring—the sense that you've successfully ushered your offspring through babyhood and on into childhood.

If overzealous breastfeeding advocates had you believing that children wean themselves after two or three years of nursing, you may feel frustrated and a little angry. Maybe you wonder if the critics of long breastfeeding have been right all along. Will your child never wean without a fight? Have you been retarding your child's social and emotional growth by letting her go on nursing? Is your child's shyness the fault of nursing? Is your relationship with your child dysfunctional? And what's wrong with you that you've developed such a relationship?

Actually, nursing still has important benefits for the child past three. For a shy child, nursing may provide the security she needs to face encounters with unfamiliar people. Nursing still soothes after upsets and injuries, comforts during illness, and makes getting to sleep easier. Some mothers say nursing after age three helps develop verbal skills, since they and their children chat together during nursing interludes. And when breastfeeding finally comes to an end for the child over three, she has the words younger children lack to talk through this developmental event.

For the mother, too, nursing past three has benefits. Many women enjoy the sociability and sensuality of breastfeeding beyond three years. This may be especially true for single mothers. A full-time worker may continue nursing to stay emotionally close to her child. Some mothers believe that the continued production of prolactin, the primary hormone involved in lactation, keeps them relaxed and patient. Besides, a child allowed to nurse to sleep at this age may continue taking naps, giving her mother an hour or two of quiet each day.

And long nursing is *natural.* In terms of species-wide behavior, you and your child are normal; it's most other Western women who are odd. Worldwide, most mothers nurse their children at least three years, and those who let their children wean themselves often nurse over five years.

Compared with other primates, too, you're normal. Katherine Dettwyler (1995) took into account gestation periods, weight gain, adult size, and age of dental eruption in species close to our own before concluding that the natural age of weaning in humans is between two and a half and seven years.

So if you've nursed your child over three years, take pride in having given her the best. But don't expect your child to initiate the end of breastfeeding—not immediately, anyway.

Self-Weaning

Children allowed to wean themselves—that is, to end breastfeeding without hints, bribes, bottles, or other encouragements—seem to do so usually between ages four and six. Although few women in our society have the patience or devotion to continue nursing long enough for their children to self-wean, those mothers who do seldom have regrets. Letting a child nurse until he feels he has nursed enough, these mothers say, fosters a lasting trust and intimacy between mother and child. Self-weaning also gives a child a sense of control and confidence; a four-year-old, when her mother asked if she would really never nurse again, smiled hugely as she replied, "No, I'm done" (Risley 1991).

Extroverted, easygoing children may give up nursing earliest and with greatest finality. Others may stop for days, weeks, or months at a time, then want to nurse again because they feel insecure, ill, or perhaps just tempted by the sight of their mothers' breasts. A boy who voluntarily gave up nursing shortly before his fifth birthday was still sucking occasionally at his mother's dry breast, for just a few minutes at a time, after he turned six.

Considering how much children love nursing, why they ever give it up voluntarily may seem a little mysterious. Some children drop nursings until eventually the milk just doesn't flow anymore. "That's all, there's no more," one child announced, and never nursed again. Another child quit nursing after complaining of headaches from sucking at a dry breast. A five-year-old explained, perhaps imaginatively, that the milk was getting too warm, and that he was trying to drink water instead.

Many children say that they're getting too old to nurse, or that nursing is a thing for babies. This happens even in families who have taken pains not to rush a child toward weaning. Children all want to grow up, and grown-ups obviously aren't nursed. But pressure to stop nursing may come from people outside the immediate family. "I really should quit," said a four-year-old, like an addict nearly ready to kick the habit. "You know, Bill quit" (Ridley 1991). Another child, a four and a half year old whose friends had teased her for nursing, couldn't openly discuss her confused feelings at first. "I don't want to nurse. . . . I hate you," she told her mother, starting to cry. When questioned, however, she explained the problem: "I want to stop and I have to hate you so I won't want to nurse anymore. I hate your breasts" (Kadushin 1977).

A child may face a difficult conflict when his friends tease him for nursing while his mother encourages him to continue. He may need his mother's reassurance that he is "a big boy" and that his mother will love him whether or not he continues to nurse. He may or may not want his mother to actively discourage him from further nursing. Either way, talking over the problem may help set a model for future parent-child communication.

Possible Reasons to Wean
Your Child Over Three

If you want to wean because your child nurses with annoying frequency or wakes you at night, or because you're pregnant, reading the sections that address these problems in Chapter 4 may give you the encouragement you need to make a guilt-free decision to stop nursing—or, instead, to find a satisfactory solution without immediately giving up nursing altogether.

Certain breastfeeding problems pertain particularly to women with nurslings over three: the fear of keeping a child dependent, the fear that you're nursing for selfish reasons, and the fear that others will accuse you of sexual abuse.

DOES LONG NURSING KEEP CHILDREN DEPENDENT?

Some older nurslings *do* seem more dependent on their mothers than the average child. Often their mothers have continued nursing only because these children reacted so anxiously to all weaning efforts. Family circumstances—such as death, divorce, frequent moves, or unhappy parents—can certainly make a child feel insecure; some women delay weaning to relieve this insecurity. But most of these late-weaning children seem to be clingy by nature. One mother explained that her daughter "always seemed to need a lot of attention, closeness, and contact. I think nursing helped fill some of those needs." Another mother summed up her child's needy disposition this way: "Give me love, give me food, give me all of you" (Owen 1989, 83).

Most older nurslings, however, are outgoing and independent, even though they may have been shy as toddlers. Many mothers, in fact, believe that their children's self-confidence, trust in others, and adventurousness—at six, eight, ten years old—are the result of long nursing. When a child's infantile needs are fulfilled, he can develop unhindered by them. Even an outgoing child may need a little extra time to grow up; as four-year-old Danny explained, "I'm still a little boy. I need mummies."

Americans tend to fear their children's dependence. Playpens, walkers, and teach-your-baby-to-read programs are all signs of our unwillingness to let babies be babies. Late development—in walking, talking, reading, weaning, or anything else—is inconvenient and embarrassing to us. Unable to fully accept the fact that human abilities develop at different rates, in each person and among different people, we wonder if the late bloomer may be suffering from a physical or mental defect. We wonder, too, if our parenting practices might be at fault. Even those of us who are home all day may feel compelled to enroll a shy child in preschool—and leave her alone there despite her cries—because we believe that this will help her to mature socially (although abandoning a child this way may actually interfere with her social maturation). The same fear provokes questions and warnings from well-meaning people about the wisdom of long breastfeeding, and drives many women to wean before their children are ready.

We should remind ourselves that the American spirit of independence, in many of its incarnations, is born not of confidence and trust but of alienation. As Elizabeth Hormann (1982) points out, "We are bent on weakening bonds in the name of growth and independence, then spend our adulthoods wondering why we have trouble getting close to other people."

Related to the fear of children's dependence is another, occasionally voiced, fear—that long nursing will promote homosexual tendencies.

Curiously, this fear is most often expressed concerning boys, not girls. This is probably because men in our society are supposed to be even more alienated than women. Keeping a little boy secure, and teaching him to appreciate intimacy, is considered feminizing. A single mother, whose son may lack the influence of a tough-talking, roughhousing dad, may face particular pressure to wean for this reason.

Your late-weaned son will likely turn out friendly and cooperative, but probably not homosexual or effeminate. In *Childhood and Society*, Erik Erikson (1963, 134-35) tells of a Sioux mother who came to school at recess to nurse her eight-year-old boy because he had a cold. This wasn't a very remarkable occurrence in her culture; the average nursing period among the Sioux, traditionally, was three to five years. Crazy Horse and Sitting Bull were probably nursed this long. These men were denounced in many ways, but never, we would bet, as emasculate.

ARE YOU NURSING FOR YOURSELF?

Certainly nursing is rewarding for most mothers—if it weren't, our species would have died out long ago. But if you nurse longer than most women in your community, others may suspect you of exploiting your child to satisfy abnormal or unhealthy needs. Sometimes you may wonder if these people are right. The nursing relationship may offer refuge from a bad marriage. It may provide solace for a mother grieving over a death in the family or a divorce. Nursing beyond three years may help to keep an older mother feeling youthful, or allow any mother who is through having children to hang on to the vestiges of her youngest child's babyhood. And long nursing may be therapeutic for a woman who was abused in childhood: Through six years of nursing her daughter, one mother said, she vicariously experienced a happy childhood, distanced herself from her abusive family of origin, and avoided becoming abusive herself.

None of these are bad reasons to continue nursing. Children of women we know in these circumstances self-weaned at four to six years, if their mothers didn't end breastfeeding first. These children weren't compelled to nurse as long as they did; most children, in fact, would nurse four to six years if allowed. In these cases long nursing is probably more protective than exploitive; it may serve to shield the child from her mother's troubles.

No one can judge better than you when it's time to wean your child. If you think you may be subconsciously prolonging nursing when your child would be better off weaned, you can try bringing nursing to a close. If your child weans without distress, you'll know she has nursed long enough. Otherwise, you needn't feel guilty about letting nursing go on a while longer.

MIGHT YOU BE ACCUSED OF CHILD ABUSE?

In numerous cases, in various parts of the United States, women have been accused of sexual abuse for nursing children over three. In an era when mass guilt about our society's treatment of children seems able to turn any parent into a suspected child abuser, some mothers worry whether long nursing may result in criminal prosecution against them or, worse, the taking of their children by governmental authorities.

In only two recent cases have children been removed from their homes because their mothers were still nursing them. The cases both involved five-year-old boys, one in Colorado and one in Illinois. In each case the child was returned to his mother, although the Illinois boy was first kept in foster care for over six months. Because both mothers were cleared of charges, the extensive publicity surrounding these cases has probably lessened the risk of prosecution for other nursing mothers. Growing support for longer breastfeeding among medical professionals may also help make such future cases unlikely.

In a 1993 article in *Mothering* magazine, Elizabeth Baldwin, a lawyer, offered advice to mothers who come under investigation for nursing children over three: Never lie; that would only make you look guilty. But don't volunteer information, either; especially, don't raise new issues by trying to explain your whole parenting style. Mentioning that you share a bed with your child, forego vaccinations, or vacation at a nudist camp might only make you more liable to harassment. If a report is filed with the police, remember your constitutional rights to remain silent and to have a lawyer present during questioning. Get a lawyer as soon as possible, and consult La Leche League for help in preparing your defense.

Katherine Dettwyler, an anthropologist who has devoted her career to the study of breastfeeding, provides a "Letter for Court Cases" in support of extended breastfeeding on her Web site. She invites mothers to send this document to legal officials, social workers, ex-spouses, and doctors; find it at www.kathydettwyler.org/detletter.htm.

This all sounds scary, we know, but remember that the risk that long breastfeeding may result in a charge of child abuse or neglect is really very small. The risk is much smaller still if you nurse your child only in private, as most children over three prefer. If charges are made, they will probably be quickly dropped. In the meantime, we hope, you will have taught some officials the lesson that long breastfeeding is not abusive at all, but is normal, healthful, and loving.

How to Wean Your Child Over Three

Weaning a child over three is relatively easy. Many women end breast-feeding through bargaining—by setting a deadline with the child or by offering a reward. Other mothers find the simplest way to stop nursing an older child is just to say no.

Many children will agree to stop nursing on their third, fourth, or fifth birthdays, at the start of preschool or kindergarten, or on another special occasion, such as the start of a long trip or their mothers' becoming pregnant. Weaning this way works best if the child is well prepared—if she is nursing no more than once or twice a day when plans are made to stop, if the deadline is set well in advance, and if the mother frequently reminds her of how soon the deadline is coming. Since reaching the deadline is a sign of the child's maturation, no other reward is usually needed; children want nothing better, after all, than to grow up. Even a child turning three may give up nursing without a word on her birthday, if the deadline is set well ahead for that day. If a child seems unprepared when her third birthday nears but her mother doesn't want to wait for the fourth, the two may settle on a half-birthday. Children who can read a bit may want to look through the calendar to choose a particular day—perhaps a holiday—a month or so in the future. Some children beat their deadlines, and take great pride in doing so.

Some mothers feel it would be unfair to take away something so precious to a child as nursing without providing something in its place. One mother weaned her five-year-old son, and later her daughter at the same age, by capitulating to their requests to buy television-advertised toys. Another mother got her son a kitten, in this way providing not only a reward for weaning, but also a substitute source of sensual pleasure.

More valuable to a child than material things may be social rewards. Following the example set in Mary Joan Deutschbein's picture book *Maggie's Weaning*, many mothers now offer their children weaning parties. Other women promise plenty of snuggling, hugging, and tickling in place of nursing. A child may finally give up the bedtime nursing if Dad agrees to read a story each night. By plan or not, most parents find themselves spending more time telling and reading stories with their children after weaning.

Some mothers just get tired of nursing and stop, often suddenly. One explained, after weaning a four-year-old this way:

I felt like I needed my body back. I was starting to cringe physically when she would nurse. I finally got disgusted enough to get really clear and firm with her. Also I realized she probably wouldn't ever stop on her own accord. That inspired me to get really strong.

Often these mothers find, to their surprise, that their children show no signs of anxiety after weaning. These mothers find that, though their children are not yet ready to wean themselves, they *are* ready to be weaned.

Not all older children are easily weaned, however. Some may be helped by the techniques of substitution and distraction (see pages 150–53). One three-year-old weaned, with difficulty, to a bottle, having never taken one before, and wouldn't give it up until three years later. Cornelia, who weaned by agreement on her fourth birthday, seemed sad and quiet for the next ten days, during which she chewed her fingernails a lot. Her mother substituted back rubs for bedtime nursings, and at nine years Cornelia still needed a back rub to get to sleep (Owen 1989, 94).

An older child who weans easily still may show some signs of loss. She may occasionally suck a thumb or finger; one five-and-a-half-year-old sucked at a small mole on her mother's collarbone and said this reminded her of her nursing days. If not permitted to nurse even momentarily after breastfeeding is formally over, a child may collapse in nervous giggles at any sight of her mother's breasts during the first few months after weaning. If allowed, a weaned child may occasionally suck briefly at the breast; one did this while pretending to be a baby lamb. Most children will find comfort, when they're tired, sick, or hurt, by placing a hand on Mama's breast.

A Lasting Gift

Whether or not a child over three occasionally nurses after weaning is formally complete, he will probably never forget how much he loved to nurse. Two years after complete weaning, five-and-a-half-year-old Andrea still pretended to nurse her dolls and talked to her mother daily about nursing. Said her mother, "She explains the feelings of being in my arms and how good it felt to nurse." Eight-and-a-half-year-old Sylvie, weaned at four, said she still missed nursing, especially the taste of the milk. Ten-year-old Kory, also weaned at four, asked a lot of questions about nursing: "Did you nurse me around other people? Did it hurt when I nursed? Did you like it, Mom?" And he is gratified when she responds honestly, "Oh, yes, it was the best time I ever had."

Life after Weaning

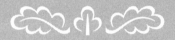

AFTER NURSING ENDS, mothers and their children experience a mix of reactions, both physical and emotional. These reactions vary greatly in kind and intensity, depending on the age and temperament of the child, how fast weaning has occurred, and how the mother has felt about breastfeeding.

Very little research has been done on women's physical reactions to weaning. For now, we must base our summary mainly on the experiences of women we know.

You will probably experience some decrease in appetite when you stop breastfeeding. Some women report losing weight and feeling restless for a week or so after weaning, but so far studies have failed to confirm that this is a common pattern. Some women, perhaps because they eat according to habit rather than appetite, gain weight after weaning.

Women normally lose 4 to 5 percent of bone density during the first three months of lactation. After weaning, normal bone density is recovered within eighteen months. These changes are governed by hormones; they occur regardless of whether a women takes supplemental calcium (Kalkwarf 1997). Still, you'll want to be sure your diet includes some calcium-rich foods. Since vitamin D is essential to calcium absorption, you'll also want to get plenty of sunshine after weaning (your baby needs sunshine, too!).

After any post-weaning engorgement and breast lumps dissipate, you will probably find that your breasts are smaller than they were before pregnancy. The areola may look shriveled, from being stretched in the baby's mouth, particularly after several years of nursing. After six months or so, new fat stores may make your breasts fill out a little.

Your breasts will probably continue to produce some fluid, if you try to express it, for months after complete weaning. Some women notice continued milk production for as long as two years after nursing ends. And, for months after the last nursing, some mothers occasionally notice the tingling sensation of milk letting down. One mother said milk leaked from her breasts during times of stress, especially when she was very worried about her child, for months after she stopped nursing.

If your periods didn't resume before the last nursing, they probably will within a few weeks—and so, probably, will your fertility. If you began menstruating before weaning was complete, expect that your next period may be early and heavy. Heavy periods may continue for several months as your body adjusts to the hormonal changes of weaning.

With the resumption of menstruation may come an increase in sex drive and vaginal lubrication (Bricklin 1987). If your periods started while you were still nursing, your sex drive may still increase at weaning, though this may be partly due to the decrease in tactile stimulation from your child. Some mothers find, however, that their breasts are less sensitive to erotic stimulation after weaning than before.

In a few women who have personal or familial histories of depression, rapid weaning in the first year may precipitate severe depression or even psychotic behavior. This may result from the hormonal changes at weaning, perhaps in combination with feelings of loss of the symbiotic mother-baby bond. Extreme anxiety, fears, frequent tearfulness, insomnia, and loss of appetite are signs that medical help is needed (Susman and Katz 1988).

Normally, a mother's feelings after weaning can vary from grief to relief. Distress after weaning is more likely the earlier weaning occurs. Some mothers, who never planned to nurse for long or who were determined not to be "tied down" by a baby, have no regrets about early weaning. But one study found that 63 percent of women who weaned at two to three months wished they could have nursed longer, and 50 percent of those who weaned at four to nine months regretted weaning so soon (Rogers, Morris, and Taper 1987).

If you have weaned before you were really ready, you may feel angry—at yourself, for not being able to do what you feel should come naturally, and at other people, perhaps for encouraging you to breastfeed, for giving inconsistent advice or none at all, or for pressuring you to wean. You may feel rejected if your baby seems to prefer the bottle to your breasts or your mate's care to your own. You may feel anxious about the baby, who is no longer getting "the best," or about your own mothering abilities. You may feel guilty about your failure to live up to your own expectations. Such feelings will be exacerbated if you had romantic visions of nursing, if you nursed an older child successfully and so feel acutely what the younger one is lacking, if you just like to do things the natural way, or if you suffered through engorgement after believing you had too little milk. If you've learned, perhaps from reading this book, that weaning wasn't necessarily the best way to solve your problems, you may feel foolish.

If you have such feelings, be assured your sadness will diminish in time. Appreciate your own courage and determination in persisting as long as you did with breastfeeding problems. Remember that any amount of breastfeeding benefits a baby, even if it's just one feeding of colostrum. Your baby will love being fed no matter what you feed her. And it *is* possible to minimize health risks and establish a strong mother-baby relationship when you must bottle-feed.

Even many mothers who breastfeed for a year or more sometimes feel sad when nursing ends. Many women speak nostalgically of the warmth, closeness, and cuddling of their nursing years. A woman may miss nursing even if she initiated weaning and has no regrets about having done so. But she is most likely to feel sad about ending nursing if her child initiated weaning. Even if the mother had planned to wean soon, she may feel surprised and a little disappointed when her child rejects her in favor of a cup or bottle.

A mother may feel guilty, too, if a child develops health problems soon after weaning. Whether or not the antibodies in her milk could have prevented the child's illness, she may regret that she can't nurse the child through the sickness. If your child gets sick soon after weaning, you might offer your breast whether or not you have any milk. Even a few weak sucks on a dry breast will probably give some solace. Your child may take comfort, too, from resting his head or hand on your breast.

Guilt feelings may also arise when a mother has weaned for what she sees as selfish reasons—to take a vacation without the kids, for instance. If the child adjusts quickly, seems happy, and is making developmental strides, guilt feelings quickly recede. But if a child regresses—to wearing diapers, for instance—or expresses unfulfilled needs in ways like thumb-sucking or carrying around a bottle, a mother may know her decision to wean was not in her child's best interests. If you find yourself in this situation, and if you can't or don't wish to start nursing again, it's probably best to allow relatively harmless self-soothing measures like thumb-sucking, but also to strive to give your child a lot of love and attention in ways such as cuddling and playing together.

Perhaps most mothers have mixed feelings about weaning when they plan to have no more children. In this case the last nursing marks the end of a woman's reproductive years. The last nursing is, like the first menstruation, a momentous life event for which our culture provides no rite of passage. Other people, even a woman's own family members, may be blind to her feelings, which she may lack words to express anyway. Perhaps this is a time to make "a great feast," as Abraham reputedly did on the day that Isaac was weaned. Both mother and child should be honored, since they have each completed a major passage from one stage of life to another.

And how do children feel after weaning? In one survey of U.S. mothers, most said their children's responses to weaning were "OK" or "happy" regardless of the children's ages (Avery 1977). Mothers elsewhere in the world have similar reports. Malian women told a researcher that their children, when suddenly weaned, weren't upset and did not cry, or cried only during the nights for a few days, and quickly forgot about nursing (Dettwyler 1987). Zulu mothers made similar assertions, although their careful preparations for weaning—planning the date months ahead, tying charms around the children's necks, spending the day at home, and in some cases even calling in a "weaning specialist," belied their apparent calm (Albino and Thompson 1956).

The Zulu women had good reason to fear, researchers found: All their children showed disturbed social behavior after weaning (see page 157). As far as we can determine, no similar studies have been made of weanlings in the United States or elsewhere. Western children might not react to weaning as strongly as Zulu children, who one day have free access to the breast and the next day have none. Still, *most* children may have stronger reactions to weaning than their parents care to talk about.

In all but a few of the Zulu children, the disturbed behavior ended within a few weeks. In describing their children after weaning, Zulu, American, and other mothers may tend to put out of their minds the stressful period immediately after nursing ends, and focus on their children's later behavior. It is not until a child has resigned herself to the loss of the breast, after all, that she can be considered fully weaned.

Some psychologists believe that no child ever resigns himself entirely to the loss of the breast. This may perhaps be true, since even children who voluntarily wean may be reacting, for instance, to a low milk supply or a sore in the mouth, and they may miss the breast even if they don't show it. In children weaned beyond about the age of three, nursing never leaves even the conscious memory, and as the older child voluntarily gives up nursing he may express ambivalence about doing so.

But as parents we must judge our children's well-being by their immediate behavior. If a child is happy and healthy now it makes no sense to worry about what he may say on a psychoanalyst's couch thirty years from now.

Our society's lack of shared standards for weaning is both a blessing and a curse. It is a curse in that it forces every mother to make the difficult decision of when and how to wean each child, and the resulting uncertainty she may feel can make weaning more of a struggle than it should be. But this lack of rules is also a blessing, in that it permits a mother to consider her child's needs over society's will. If a child is anxious, clingy, and sad during gradual weaning or soon after the last nursing, the mother can always start nursing again, at least as often as is necessary for her child's comfort.

Whether or not they are willing to postpone complete weaning, most mothers go out of their way to make up for the end of breastfeeding. They may be tempted to use the time no longer spent nursing in activities that exclude the child, but just-weaned children usually demand a lot of atten- tion. After weaning a mother usually finds herself in a transformed but still demanding relationship with her child. Feeding a baby with a bottle, cup, or spoon is hard work, as are the talking, playing, reading, and com- forting that a toddler or older child demands. The effort pays off, moth- ers find, as their weaned children venture into the world, making developmental strides in such areas as walking and talking, and perhaps becoming more independent, outgoing, and responsible. When these things happens, a mother knows her child has put any anger or sadness about weaning behind her; she is truly well weaned.

APPENDIX

Positioning and Latch-on Techniques

The cross-over hold is one of two positions in which you can most easily get your young baby to latch on to the breast. Compared with the cradle hold, in which the baby's head rests in the bend of the elbow, the cross-over hold gives you more control over his head when you pull him onto the breast.

To begin, sit in a comfortable chair with arms. The chair should allow you to sit up straight; most couches are too deep. Place one or two pillows on your lap so that the baby is at the level of the breast. Turn the baby so that his tummy is against yours. Instead of holding the baby's head in the bend of your elbow, as in the cradle hold, hold him with the opposite arm, so that your hand supports the back of his head. For maximum support and control of the baby's head, place your thumb behind and just below one ear and the other fingers behind and just below the other. Position the baby's face directly in front of your breast, so you won't have to push the breast sideways toward the baby.

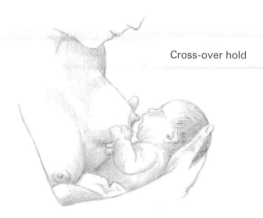

Cross-over hold

Imagine you have a clock face stamped on each breast. If you're starting on the right breast, hold the breast with the right hand so that your thumb is positioned about 1½ inches from the nipple at nine o'clock and your index finger the same distance from the nipple at three o'clock. Compress the areola with your thumb and index finger. This U-shaped hold with compression will more closely match your breast to the shape of the baby's mouth so he can take in more of the breast.

With the baby and breast in position and the baby's nose in front of the nipple, touch the baby's upper lip to your nipple until he opens his mouth wide. At the moment that his mouth is wide open, quickly bring

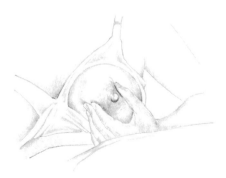

Hand position for the cross-over hold

the baby onto the breast, chin first, keeping the areola compressed until the baby begins sucking. Avoid three mistakes that new mothers commonly make: aligning the baby's mouth rather than his nose with the nipple, not pulling the baby on far enough, and releasing the areola before the baby is well latched on.

Another position that lets you clearly see what you're doing and control the process of latching on is the *football hold.* This is usually the hold of choice for women with large breasts. To begin, sit in a comfortable chair with arms. Place a pillow to your side, between you and the arm of the chair. Place the baby on the pillow facing the back of the chair, and support her in a semi-sitting position facing the back of the chair. Your arm should support her back, and your hand should hold her head. Place your thumb behind one ear and the other fingers behind the other. The top of the baby's head should be as high as the top of your breast.

Support your breast with your free hand so that your thumb is about 1½ inches behind the nipple at twelve o'clock and your index finger is the same distance from the nipple at six o'clock. Compress the areola with your thumb and index finger. This C-shaped hold with compression will more closely match your breast to the shape of the baby's mouth so she can take in more of the breast.

As with the cross-over hold, stimulate the baby to open wide, bring her onto the breast, and then release the areola.

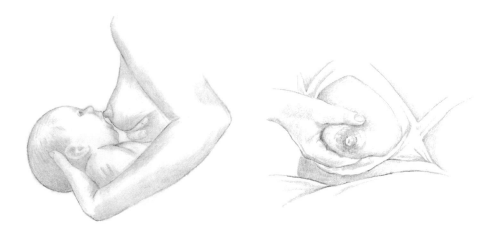

Football hold and hand position

Breastfeeding Support Groups

La Leche League International
P.O. Box 4079
Schaumburg, Illinois 60168
800-LA-LECHE or 847-519-7730
www.lalecheleague.org

Call weekdays between 9:00 A.M. and 3:00 P.M. Central Standard
Time for breastfeeding help or a referral to a local La Leche leader or
group. Or check the white pages of your phone book; most list a local
La Leche League leader's phone number under "La Leche League."

Boston Association for Childbirth Education (BACE)
Nursing Mothers' Council
P.O Box 29
Newtonville, Massachusetts 02460
617-244-5102
www.bace-nmc.org

Nursing Mothers' Counsel, Inc.
P.O. Box 50063
Palo Alto, California 94303
408-291-8008
www.nursingmothers.org

There are three chapters in Northern California (San Francisco–San
Mateo, Santa Cruz, and Santa Clara counties).

Lactation Professional Referral Services

International Lactation Consultant Association
1500 Sunday Drive, Suite 102
Raleigh, North Carolina 27607
919-861-5577
E-mail: info@ilca.org
www.ilca.org

International Board of Lactation Consultant Examiners (IBLCE)
7245 Arlington Boulevard, Suite 200
Falls Church, Virginia 22042
703-560-7330
E-mail: iblce@iblce.org
www.iblce.org

Breastfeeding National Network (Medela, Inc.)
800-TELL-YOU or 800-435-8316
www.medela.com/NEWFILES/bnn.html

Call at any hour for referral to a local lactation consultant.

Electric Breast Pump Rental Companies

Medela, Inc.
P.O. Box 660
McHenry, Illinois 60051
800-TELL-YOU or 800-435-8316
www.medela.com

Medela's Breastfeeding National Network can refer you to a local
rental station, where you can rent either a full-sized electric pump or
the more portable Lactina Plus, a lightweight, fully automatic pump
that has an optional adapter for a battery pack or cigarette lighter.
Call at any hour.

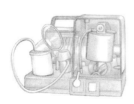 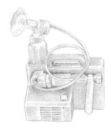

Full-sized electric pump (left) and Lactina Plus electric pump

Hollister Ameda Breastfeeding Products
2000 Hollister Drive
Libertyville, Illinois 60048
800-323-4060
www.hollister.com

Call weekdays between 8:00 A.M. and 5:00 P.M.
Central Standard Time to locate a Hollister pump.

Breast Shells

LilyPadz
Me & My Kidz
P.O. Box 27346
Macon, Georgia 31221
www.lilypadz.com

Medela Soft Shells and TheraShells
Medela, Inc.
P.O. Box 660
McHenry, Illinois 60051
800-435-8316
www.medela.com

Nursing Supplementer

Supplemental Nursing System
Medela, Inc.
P.O. Box 660
McHenry, Illinois 60051
800-435-8316
www.medela.com

Information about Drugs in Breast Milk

U.C.S.D. Drug Information Service
University of California, San Diego
619-543-6971

Call Monday through Friday between 9:00 A.M. and 5:00 P.M. Pacific Standard Time with questions about drugs and breastfeeding.

LactMed database of drugs and breastfeeding
National Library of Medicine
toxnet.nlm.nih.gov/cgi-bin/sis/htmlgen?LACT

REFERENCES

Abrams, C., et al. 1975. "Hazards of Overconcentrated Milk Formula." *Journal of the American Medical Association 232*: 1136-40.

Alalussa, Satu, et al. 1990. "Prevalence of Caries and Salivary Levels of Mutans Streptococci in 5-Year-Old Children in Relation to Duration of Breast Feeding." *Scandinavian Journal of Dental Research 98:* 193-96.

Albino, Ronald C., and V. J. Thompson. 1956. "The Effects of Sudden Weaning on Zulu Children." *Medical Psychology 29:* 177-210.

Aloia, J. F. et al. 1985. "Risk Factors in Postmenopausal Osteoporosis." *American Journal of Medicine 78:* 95-100.

Aniansson, G., et al. 1994. "A Prospective Cohort Study on Breast-feeding and Otitis Media in Swedish Infants." *Pediatric Infectious Disease Journal 13:* 183-88.

Apple, Rima. 1987. *Mothers and Medicine: A Social History of Infant Feeding, 1890-1950.* Madison: University of Wisconsin Press.

_____. 1992. "The Role of the Medical Profession in Promoting Artificial Feeding." Lecture presented at the 1992 International Lactation Consultant Association Annual Meeting and Conference, Chicago, Illinois.

Arnon, S. S. 1986. "Infant Botulism: Anticipating the Second Decade." *Journal of Infectious Diseases 154:* 201-6.

Bahna, S. L. 1987. "Milk Allergy in Infancy." *Annals of Allergy 59:* 131-36.

Baldwin, Elizabeth N. 1993. "Extended Breastfeeding and the Law." *Mothering* (Spring): 88–91.

_____. 2001. "Extended Breastfeeding and the Law." *Breastfeeding Abstracts* 20: 19–20.

Ball, Thomas M., and Anne L. Wright. 1999. "Health Care Costs of Formula-feeding in the First Year of Life." *Pediatrics 103:* 870-76.

Bauer, G., et al. 1991. "Breastfeeding and Cognitive Development of Three-Year-Old Children." *Psychological Reports 68:* 1218.

Bener, A., et al. 2001. "Longer Breastfeeding and Protection against Childhood Leukemia and Lymphomas." *European Journal of Cancer 37:* 234-38.

Bishop, N., M. McGraw, and N. Ward. 1989. "Aluminum in Infant Formulas." *Lancet* 2 (8637): 490.

Brazelton, T. Berry. 1983. *Infants and Mothers: Differences in Development.* Rev. ed. New York: Delta/Seymour Lawrence.

Broad, F. E., and D. M. Duganzich. 1983. "The Effects of Infant Feeding, Birth Order, Occupation, and Socio-Economic Status on Speech in Six-Year-Old Children." *New Zealand Medical Journal 96:* 483-6.

Brock, K. E., et al. 1989. "Sexual, Reproductive, and Contraceptive Risk Factors for Carcinoma-In-Situ for the Uterine Cervix in Sydney." *Medical Journal of Australia 150:* 125-30.

Bronson, G. 1980. "Breastfeeding Advocates Increasingly Question Safety, Nutritional Value of Infants' Formula." *Wall Street Journal* (Friday, March 20): 40.

Buckley, Kathleen M. 1992. "Beliefs and Practices Related to Extended Breastfeeding among La Leche League Mothers." *Journal of Perinatal Education 1:* 45-53.

Bumgarner, Norma Jane. 2000. *Mothering Your Nursing Toddler.* Franklin Park, Illinois: La Leche League International.

Byers, T., et al. 1985. "Lactation and Breast Cancer. Evidence for a Negative Association in Pre-menopausal Women." *American Journal of Epidemiology 121:* 664-74.

Cable, Thomas A., and Lee A. Rothenberger. 1984. "Breast-Feeding Behavioral Patterns among La Leche League Mothers: A Descriptive Survey." *Pediatrics 73:* 830-35.

Clark, S., and R. Harmon. 1983. "Infant-Initiated Weaning from the Breast in the First Year." *Early Human Development 8:* 151-56.

Cochi, S. L., et al. 1986. "Primary Invasive Haemophilus Influenza Type B Disease: A Population-based Assessment of Risk Factors." *Journal of Pediatrics 108:* 887-96.

Collipp, P. J., S. Y. Chen, and S. Maitinsky. 1983. "Manganese in Infant Formula and Learning Disability." *Annals of Nutrition and Metabolism 27:* 488-94.

Curzon, M. E. J., and K. J. Toumba. 1997. "Plumbing the Depths of Dental Decay." *Nature Medicine 3:* 956.

Dagnelie, P. C., et al. 1989. "Nutritional Status of Infants Age 4 to 18 Months on Macrobiotic Diets and Matched Omnivorous Control Infants: A Population-Based Mixed-Longitudinal Study." *European Journal of Clinical Nutrition 43:* 311-23.

Davis, Clara M. 1928. "Self-Selection of Diets in Newly Weaned Infants." *American Journal of Diseases of Children 36:* 651-79.

Davis, M. K., D. A. Savitz, and B. I. Graubard. 1988. "Infant Feeding and Childhood Cancer." *Lancet 2* (8607): 365-68.

Dettwyler, Katherine A. 1987. "Breastfeeding and Weaning in Mali: Cultural Context and Hard Data." *Social Science Medicine 24:* 633-44.

_____. 1995. "A Time to Wean: The Hominid Blueprint for the Natural Age of Weaning in Modern Human Populations." In *Breastfeeding: Biocultural Perspectives,* edited by P. Stuart-Macadam and K. A. Dettwyler. New York: Aldine de Gruyter, 305-45.

_____. 2005. "Letter for Court Cases (in Support of Extended Breastfeeding)." www.kathydettwyler.org/detletter.htm.

Dettwyler, K. A., K. G. Dewey, A. D. Findley, and B. Lonnerdale. 1984. "Breast Milk Volume and Composition during Late Lactation (7-20 Months)." *Journal of Pediatric Gastroenterological Nutrition* 3: 713-20.

Deutschbein, Mary Joan. 1999. *Maggie's Weaning.* Schaumburg, Illinois: La Leche League International.

Dewey, K. G., M. J. Heinig, and L. A. Nommsen. 1993. "Maternal Weight-Loss Patterns during Prolonged Lactation." *American Journal of Clinical Nutrition 58:* 162-66.

Dorner, G., and H. Grychtolik. 1978. "Long-Lasting Ill-Effects of Neonatal Qualitative and/or Quantitative Dysnutrition in the Human." *Endokrinologie 71:* 81-88.

Duncan, B., et al. 1993. "Exclusive Breast-feeding for at Least 4 Months Protects Against Otitis Media." *Pediatrics 91:* 867-72.

Elias, Marjorie F., et al. 1986. "Sleep/Wake Patterns of Breastfed Infants in the First 2 Years of Life." *Pediatrics 77:* 322-29.

Erickson, P. R., and E. Mazhari. 1999. "Investigation of the Role of Human Breast Milk in Caries Development." *Pediatric Dentistry 21*: 86-90.

Erikson, Erik H. 1963. *Childhood and Society,* 2nd ed. New York: W. W. Norton.

Fackelmann, Kathy A. 1992. "Motherhood and Cancer." *Science News 142:* 298-300.

Fallot, M. E., J. L. Boyd, and F. A. Oski. 1980. "Breastfeeding Reduces Incidence of Hospital Admissions for Infections in Infants." *Pediatrics 65:* 1121-24.

Feachem, R. G., and M. A. Koblinsky. 1984. "Interventions for the Control of Diarrhoeal Diseases among Young Children: Promotion of Breastfeeding." *Bulletin of the World Health Organization 62:* 271-91.

Ferber, Richard. 2006. *Solve Your Child's Sleep Problems: The Complete Practical Guide for Parents.* Rev. ed. New York: Simon and Schuster.

Fergusson, D. M., A. L. Beautrais, and P. A. Silva. 1982. "Breastfeeding and Cognitive Development in the First Seven Years of Life." *Social Science Medicine 16:* 1705-8.

Fildes, Valerie A. 1986. *Breasts, Bottles, and Babies: A History of Infant Feeding.* Edinburgh: Edinburgh University Press.

Fisher, D. 1989. "Upper Limit of Iodine in Infant Formula." *Journal of Nutrition 119:* 1865-68.

Ford, R. P. K., et al. 1993. "Breastfeeding and the Risk of Sudden Infant Death Syndrome." *International Journal of Epidemiology 22:* 885-99.

Frederickson, D. D., et al. 1993. "Relationship of Sudden Infant Death Syndrome to Breast-Feeding Duration and Intensity." *American Journal of Diseases of Children 147:* 460.

Garza, Cuberto, et al. 1983. "Changes in the Nutrient Composition of Human Milk during Gradual Weaning." *American Journal of Clinical Nutrition 37:* 61-65.

Goldman, A. S., R. M. Goldblum, and C. Garza. 1983. "Immunologic Components of Human Milk during the Second Year of Lactation." *Acta Paediatrica Scandanavica 72:* 461-62.

Gordon, Jay, and Maria Goodavage. 2002. *Good Nights: The Happy Parents' Guide to the Family Bed (and a Peaceful Night's Sleep!).* New York: St. Martin's Griffin.

Greco, L., et al. 1988. "Case-Control Study on Nutritional Risk Factors in Celiac Disease." *Journal of Pediatric Gastroenterology and Nutrition 7:* 395-99.

Gwinn, M. L., et al. 1990. "Pregnancy, Breastfeeding, and Oral Contraceptives and the Risk of Epithelial Ovarian Cancer." *Journal of Clinical Epidemiology 43:* 559-68.

Habbick, B. K., C. Khanna, and T. To. 1989. "Infantile Hypertrophic Pyloric Stenosis: A Case Study of Feeding Practices and Other Possible Causes." *Canadian Medical Association Journal 140:* 401-4.

Hahn-Zoric, M., et al. 1990. "Antibody Responses to Parenteral and Oral Vaccines Are Impaired by Conventional and Low-Protein Formulas as Compared to Breastfeeding." *Acta Paediatrica Scandanavica 79:* 1137-42.

Harder, Thomas. 2005. "Duration of Breastfeeding and Risk of Overweight: A Meta-Analysis." *American Journal of Epidemiology 162* (5): 397-403.

Heinig, M. J., et al. 1994. "Factors Related to Duration of Postpartum Amenorrhoea among USA Women with Prolonged Lactation." *Journal of Biosocial Science 26:* 517-27.

Hervada, Arturo R., and Debra R. Newman. 1992. "Weaning: Historical Perspectives, Practical Recommendations, and Current Controversies." *Current Problems in Pediatrics 5:* 223-40.

Ho, M., et al. 1988. "Diarrheal Deaths in American Children: Are They Preventable?" *Journal of the American Medical Association 260:* 3281-85.

Hormann, Elizabeth. 1982. "Prolonged Nursing." *Mothering* (Spring): 70-73.

Horwood, J. L., and D. M. Fergusson. 1998. "Breastfeeding and Later Cognitive and Academic Outcomes." *Pediatrics 101:* 9.

Huggins, Kathleen. 2005. *The Nursing Mother's Companion*, 5th ed. Boston: Harvard Common Press.

Huggins, Kathleen, and Sharon Billon. 1993. "Twenty Cases of Persistent Sore Nipples: Collaboration Between Lactation Consultant and Dermatologist." *Journal of Human Lactation 9:* 155-60.

"Inadequate Vegan Diets at Weaning." 1990. *Nutrition Reviews 48:* 323-26.

Ivarsson, A., et al. 2002. "Breast-feeding Protects against Celiac Disease." *American Journal of Clinical Nutrition 75:* 914-21.

Ivarsson, A., et al. 2000. "Epidemic of Coeliac Disease in Swedish Children." *Acta Paediatrica 89:* 165-71.

Jackson, Deborah. 2003. *Three in a Bed.* London: Bloomsbury.

Jakobsson, I., and T. Lindberg. 1983. "Cow's Milk Proteins Cause Infantile Colic in Breast-fed Infants: A Double-Blind Crossover Study." *Pediatrics 71:* 268-71.

Jefferis, G. G., and A. M. Nichols. 1894. *The Household Guide or Domestic Cyclopedia, Home Remedies for Man and Beast,* 13th ed., 124-32. Reprinted in *Journal of Human Lactation 8* (1992): 93-95.

Jensen, Rima. 1992. "Fenugreek—Overlooked But Not Forgotten." *UCLA Lactation Alumni Association Newsletter 1:* 2-3.

Kadushin, Adrianne. 1977. "Breastfeeding and Weaning the Preschool Child." *Keeping Abreast Journal* (July–September): 208-11.

Kalwarf, H. J., et al. 1997. "The Effects of Calcium Supplementation on Bone Density during Lactation and after Weaning." *New England Journal of Medicine 337:* 558-59.

Kandhai, M. C., et al. 2004. "Occurrence of *Enterobacter sakazakii* in Food Production Environments and Households." *Lancet 363:* 39-40.

Kennedy, Kathy, et al. 1989. "Consensus Statement on the Use of Breastfeeding as a Family Planning Method." *Contraception 39:* 477-96.

Kennedy, K. I., and C. M. Visness. 1992. "Contraceptive Efficacy of Lactational Amenorrhoea." *Lancet 339:* 227-230.

Koetting, C. A., and G. M. Wardlaw. 1988. "Wrist, Spine, and Hip Bone Density in Women with Variable Histories of Lactation." *American Journal of Clinical Nutrition 48:* 1479-81.

Koletzko, S., et al. 1989. "Role of Infant Feeding Practices in Development of Crohn's Disease in Childhood." *British Medical Journal* 298: 1617-18.

Labbok, M. H., and G. E. Hendershot. 1987. "Does Breastfeeding Protect Against Malocclusion? Analysis of the 1981 Child Health Supplement to the National Health Interview Survey." *American Journal of Preventative Medicine 3:* 227-32.

Lawrence, Ruth A. 2005. *Breastfeeding: A Guide for the Medical Profession.* 6th ed. St. Louis: Elsevier/C. V. Mosby.

Layde, P. M., et al. 1989. "The Independent Associations of Parity, Age of First Full-Term Pregnancy, and Duration of Breastfeeding with the Risk of Breast Cancer." *Journal of Clinical Epidemiology 42:* 963-73.

Lewis, P. R., et al. 1991. "The Resumption of Ovulation and Menstruation in a Well-Nourished Population of Women Breastfeeding for an Extended Period of Time." *Fertility and Sterility 55:* 529-36.

Lonnerdal, B., C. A. Lovelady, and K. G. Dewey. 1990. "Lactation Performance of Exercising Women." *American Journal of Clinical Nutrition 52:* 103-9.

Lozoff, B., et al. 1987. "Iron Deficiency Anemia and Iron Therapy Effects on Infant Development and Test Performance." *Pediatrics 79:* 981-95.

Lucas, A., et al. 1992. "Breastmilk and Subsequent Intellegence Quotient in Children Born Preterm." *Lancet 339:* 261-64.

Luotonen, M., et al. 1996. "Recurrent Otitis Media during Infancy and Linguistic Skills at the Age of Nine Years." *Pediatric Infectious Disease Journal 15:* 854-58.

Maclean, Heather. 1990. *Women's Experience of Breastfeeding.* Toronto: University of Toronto Press.

Mandel, D., et al. 2005. "Fat and Energy Contents of Expressed Human Breast Milk in Prolonged Lactation." *Pediatrics 116:* 432-35.

Mayer, E. J., et al. 1988. "Reduced Risk of IDDM among Breastfed Children." *Diabetes 37:* 1625-32.

McJunkin, J. E., W. G. Bithoney, and M. C. McCormick. 1987. "Errors in Formula Concentration in an Outpatient Population." *Journal of Pediatrics 111:* 848-50.

McTiernan, A., and D. B. Thomas. 1986. "Evidence for a Protective Effect of Lactation on Risk of Breast Cancer in Young Women." *American Journal of Epidemiology 124:* 353-58.

Melton, L. J., et al. 1993. "Influence of Breastfeeding and Other Reproductive Factors on Bone Mass Later in Life." *Osteoporosis International 3:* 76-83.

Merrett, T. G., et al. 1988. "Infant Feeding and Allergy: Twelve Month Prospective Study of 500 Babies Born in Allergic Families." *Annals of Allergy 61:* 13-20.

Mitchell, E. A., et al. 1991. "Cot Death Supplement: Results from the First Year of the New Zealand Cot Death Study." *New Zealand Medical Journal 104:* 71-76.

Morley, R., et al. 1988. "Mother's Choice to Provide Breastmilk and Developmental Outcome." *Archives of Disease in Childhood 63:* 1382-85.

Morrow-Tlucak, M., R. H. Haude, and C. B. Ernhart. 1988. "Breastfeeding and Cognitive Development in the First Two Years of Life." *Social Science Medicine 26:* 635-39.

Morse, Janice M., and Margaret J. Harrison. 1987. "Social Coercion for Weaning." *Journal of Nurse-Midwifery 32:* 205-10.

Moscone, S. R., and M. J. Moore. 1993. "Breastfeeding during Pregnancy." *Journal of Human Lactation 9:* 83-88.

Newman, Jack. 1993. "The Bottle Feeding Mindset: How It Develops and Affects Breastfeeding." Lecture presented at the 1993 International Lactation Consultant Association Annual Meeting and Conference, Phoenix, Arizona.

Newton, N., and M. Theotokatos. 1979. "Breastfeeding during Pregnancy in 503 Women: Does a Psychobiological Weaning Mechanism Exist in Humans?" In *Emotion and Reproduction,* edited by L. Zichella. London: Academic Press, 845-49.

Owen, Siena Klein. 1989. *Weaning Ways: A Collection of Mothers' Nursing and Weaning Experiences.* Garberville, California: Shared Experiences Publishing.

Pantley, Elizabeth. 2002. *The No-Cry Sleep Solution.* New York: Contemporary Books.

Pinczuk, Jane M. 1998. *Michele, the Nursing Toddler.* Schaumburg, Illinois: La Leche International.

Pisacane, A., et al. 1992. "Breastfeeding and Urinary Tract Infections." *Journal of Pediatrics 120:* 87-89.

Popkin, B. M., et al. 1990. "Breast-feeding and Diarrheal Morbidity." *Pediatrics 86:* 874-82.

Rickert, V. I., and C. Merle Johnson. 1988. "Reducing Nocturnal Awakening and Crying Episodes in Infants and Young Children: A Comparison Between Scheduled Awakenings and Systematic Ignoring." *Pediatrics 81:* 203-12.

Riordan, J., and F. Nichols. 1990. "A Descriptive Study of Lactation Mastitis in Long-Term Breastfeeding Women." *Journal of Human Lactation 6:* 53-58.

Ripa, Louis W. 1988. "Nursing Caries: A Comprehensive Review." *Pediatric Dentistry 10:* 268-82.

Rogers, Cosby S., Sandra Morris, and L. Janette Taper. 1987. "Weaning from the Breast: Influences on Maternal Decisions." *Pediatric Nursing 13:* 341-45.

Ross, Louise. 1981. "Weaning Practices." *Journal of Nurse-Midwifery 26:* 9-14.

Rossiter, Frederick M. 1908. *The Practical Guide to Health, A Popular Treatise on Anatomy, Physiology, and Hygiene, with a Scientific*

Description of Diseases, Their Causes and Treatment Designed for Nurses and for Home Use, 462-63, 500-6, 508. Washington: Review and Herald Publishing. Reprinted in *Journal of Human Lactation 7* (1991): 89-91.

Ryan, Alan S. 1997. "The Resurgence of Breastfeeding in the United States." *Pediatrics 99:* 12.

Saarinen, U. M. 1982. "Prolonged Breastfeeding as Prophylaxis for Recurrent Otitis Media." *Acta Paediatrica Scandanavica 71:* 567-71.

Satter, Ellyn. 2000. *Child of Mine: Feeding with Love and Good Sense.* 3rd ed. Palo Alto: Bull Publishing.

Scariati, P. D., et al. 1997. "A Longitudinal Analysis of Infant Morbidity and the Extent of Breastfeeding in the United States." *Pediatrics 99:* e5.

Schachter, Frances Fuchs, et al. 1989. "Co-sleeping and Sleep Problems in Hispanic-American Urban Young Children." *Pediatrics 84:* 522-30.

Schilder, A. G. M., et al. 1993. "Long-term Effects of Otitis Media with Effusion on Language, Reading and Spelling." *Clinical Otolaryngology and Allied Sciences 18:* 234-41.

Shannon, M. W., and J. W. Graf. 1992. "Lead Intoxication in Infancy." *Pediatrics 89:* 87-90.

Sheikh, C., and P. R. Erickson. 1996. "Evaluation of Plaque pH Changes Following Oral Rinse with Eight Infant Formulas." *Pediatric Dentistry 18:* 200-204.

Shu, X. O., et al. "Infant Breastfeeding and the Risk of Childhood Lymphoma and Leukaemia." *International Journal of Epidemiology 24:* 27-32.

Simmons, B. P., et al. 1989. "*Enterbacter sakazakii* Infections in Neonates Associated with Intrinsic Contamination of a Powdered Infant Formula." *Infection Control and Hospital Epidemiology 10:* 398-401.

Smith, Betty. 1943. *A Tree Grows in Brooklyn.* Philadelphia: Blakiston Company.

Stern, J. M., et al. 1986. "Nursing Behavior, Prolactin, and Post-Partum Amenorrhea during Prolonged Lactation in American and Kung Mothers." *Clinical Endocrinology 25:* 247-58.

Susman, Virginia L., and Jack L. Katz. 1988. "Weaning and Depression: Another Postpartum Complication." *American Journal of Psychiatry 145:* 498-501.

Tanoue, Y., and S. Oda. 1989. "Weaning Time of Children with Infantile Autism." *Journal of Autism and Development Disorders 19:* 425-34.

Taylor, B., and J. Wadsworth. 1984. "Breastfeeding and Child Development at Five Years." *Developmental Medicine and Child Neurology 26:* 37-80.

Teele, D. W., et al. 1990. "Otitis Media in Infancy and Intellectual Ability, School Achievement, Speech, and Language at Age 7 Years." *Journal of Infectious Diseases 162:* 685-94.

Tully, Julia, and Kathryn G. Dewey. 1985. "Private Fears, Global Loss: A Cross-Cultural Study of the Insufficient Milk Syndrome." *Medical Anthropology 9:* 225-43.

Verdi, Tullio Suzzara. 1873. *Maternity: A Popular Treatise for Young Wives and Mothers.* New York: J. B. Ford and Co. Reprinted in *Journal of Human Lactation 5* (1989): 138-41.

Waletsky, Lucy R. 1977. "Weaning from the Breast." *World Journal of Psychosynthesis 9:* 10-14.

Walker, Marsha. 1992. "Why Aren't More Mothers Breastfeeding?" *Childbirth Educator 2* (1) 19-27.

_____. 1993a. "A Fresh Look at the Risks of Artificial Infant Feeding." *Journal of Human Lactation 9:* 97-107.

_____. 1993b. "Hazards of Infant Formula: Update." Lecture presented at the 1993 International Lactation Consultant Association Annual Meeting and Conference, Phoenix, Arizona.

Watson, G. E., et al. 1997. "Influence of Maternal Lead Ingestion on Caries in Rat Pups." *Nature Medicine 3:* 1024.

Wertz, Richard W., and Dorothy C. Wertz. 1979. *Lying-In: A History of Childbirth in America.* New York: Schocken Books.

Whiting, John W. M., and Irvin L. Child. 1953. *Child Training and Personality: A Cross-Cultural Study.* New Haven: Yale University Press.

Wickes, Ian G. 1953. "A History of Infant Feeding." *Archives of Diseases of Childhood 28:* 151-58, 332-40, 416-22, 495-501.

Williams, K. M., and Janice M. Morse, 1989. "Weaning Patterns of First-Time Mothers." *American Journal of Maternal/Child Nursing 14:* 188-92.

Woolridge, M. W., and C. Fisher. 1988. "Colic, 'Overfeeding,' and Symptoms of Lactose Malabsorption in the Breast-fed Baby: A Possible Artifact of Feed Management?" *Lancet* 2 (8607) : 382-84.

Wright, A. L., et al. 1989. "Breastfeeding and Lower Respiratory Tract Illness in the First Year of Life." *British Medical Journal 299*: 946-49.

Wright, A. L., et al. 1995. "Relationship of Infant Feeding to Recurrent Wheezing at Age 6 Years." *Archives of Pediatrics and Adolescent Medicine 149:* 758-63.

Wright, Anne L., and Richard J. Schanler. 2001. "The Resurgence of Breastfeeding at the End of the Second Millennium." *Journal of Nutrition 131:* 421S-25S.

Zheng, Tongzhang, et al. 2000. "Lactation Reduces Breast Cancer Risk in Shandong Province, China." *American Journal of Epidemiology 152:* 1129-35.

Ziegler, E. E., et al. 1990. "Cow Milk Feeding in Infancy: Further Observations on Blood Loss from the Gastrointestinal Tract." *Journal of Pediatrics 116:* 11-18.

INDEX